PRAISE FOR THE FIRST EDIT

Nursing Mother, Working Mother

"I wish I had written this easy-to-read and empowering book. Pryor makes clear *how,* not just why, a mother will combine breastfeeding and paid employment. A 'must read' for any woman considering such a combination of experiences."
–Kathleen Auerbach, PhD, IBCLC, Private Lactation Consultant

"A practical guide to resolving some of the difficulties that can occur when a breastfeeding mother returns to her job after maternity leave." —*Los Angeles Times*

"Sensitive, insightful guide." —*Booklist*

"Resourceful, confidence-building text." —*Publishers Weekly*

"A highly practical yet philosophical book that will empower mothers." —*Library Journal*

"A fine addition to the reading list of any new mother hoping to balance mothering and a professional or business career."
—*Journal of the Association for Research on Mothering*

"A terrific and detailed guide on how to nurse your baby and go back to work at the same time. This book is a refreshing, candid look the demands a working mother faces today."
—*Childbirth Instructor*

"Gale Pryor has drawn from her breastfeeding experiences while working full-time to produce a book that will prove extremely useful to women experiencing frequent separations from their breastfed babies ... provides a wealth of knowledge on the practical aspects of breastfeeding."
—La Leche League International's *New Beginnings* magazine

"With the sensitivity of a mother who has 'been there,' Pryor gives the reader confidence and reassurance that combining breastfeeding and working is possible and provides ample suggestions to back it up ... I strongly recommend every mother read it." —Gail Martel, *Journal of Human Lactation*

"Full of practical hints on overcoming social and workplace obstacles to breastfeeding." *—Fit Pregnancy*

"Empowers women who desire to blend their roles of motherhood with a job outside the home in a confident and successful way." *—The Journal of Perinatal and Neonatal Nursing*

"Gale Pryor writes an in-depth and passionate book for and about the nursing, working mother. Not only is it very supportive of working women, but it also provides the basic information needed for any woman to successfully breastfeed her baby." *—Journal of the Section on Women's Health*

"*Nursing Mother, Working Mother* provides a road map for successful mothering. In a graceful tone of respect and understanding, Gale Pryor offers detailed and practical advice so that every mother who wants to can return to work with confidence that she and her baby will maintain their special intimacy."
—Bettyann Holtzmann Kevles, author of
*Naked to the Bone: Medical
Imaging in the Twentieth Century*

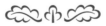

Nursing Mother, Working Mother

Nursing Mother, Working Mother

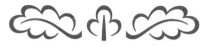

The Essential Guide to
Breastfeeding Your Baby
Before and After
You Return to Work

SECOND EDITION

GALE PRYOR AND KATHLEEN HUGGINS, R.N., M.S.

THE HARVARD COMMON PRESS
BOSTON, MASSACHUSETTS

The Harvard Common Press
535 Albany Street
Boston, Massachusetts 02118
www.harvardcommonpress.com

Printed in the United States of America
Printed on acid-free paper

Library of Congress Cataloging-in-Publication Data

Pryor, Gale.
   Nursing mother, working mother : the essential guide to breastfeeding
your baby before and after you return to work / Gale Pryor and Kathleen
Huggins.—2nd ed.
      p. cm.
   Includes bibliographical references and index.
   ISBN 1-55832-331-7 (pbk. : alk. paper)
   1. Breastfeeding—Popular works. 2. Working mothers. I. Huggins,
Kathleen. II. Title.
   RJ216.P768 2006
   649'.33—dc22

                                                        2006026173

                        978-1-55832-331-5

Special bulk-order discounts are available on this and other
Harvard Common Press books. Companies and organizations may
purchase books for premiums or resale, or may arrange a custom
edition, by contacting the Marketing Director at the address above.

BOOK DESIGN BY JILL WEBER

COVER ILLUSTRATION BY COCO MASUDA

ILLUSTRATIONS BY ALEXIS SEABROOK

10 9 8 7 6 5 4 3 2

For my boys:
Kolya, Max, Wylie, and Nathaniel
—G.P.

To John, my baby boy whom
I nursed while I worked.
—K.H.

CONTENTS

ACKNOWLEDGMENTS

THIS BOOK BEGAN TAKING SHAPE when I returned to work following the birth of my first son, Max. In a new city far from family, the first among my friends to become a mother, unique among my coworkers in attempting to combine mothering and working, I was overwhelmed by anxiety and strain. The support of experienced mothers and friends in the same stage of life would have made everything so much easier.

At the very least, a book that addressed my situation, including both the practical problems to which I was devising answers and the emotional events I was weathering, would have helped a great deal. Now, having authored that wished-for book, I know that having a baby and writing a book share much in common: friends and family make the job so much easier.

Neither my sons nor this book would have been possible without the help of my best friend and husband, Karl Leabo. His encouragement as I spent hours upon hours at the computer, his gift of a beautiful desk, his endless patience at living with piles of papers, boxes of books, and ink stains on the bed sheets whenever I fell asleep while underlining a reference were all major contributions to the completion of the writing. The imaginative weekend expeditions on which he took our sons, while I stayed home to write, vastly improved what could have been a dreary year for them. These sons, Max, Wylie, and Nathaniel (who came along in time for the second edition), deserve thanks as well. They have been my inspiration, my teachers, and my rewards throughout the hard work of becoming a mother and a writer.

This book also came to be because of my mother, Karen Pryor. Writer, biologist, behaviorist, breastfeeding expert, dolphin researcher, dog guru, keynote speaker, grandmother, birdwatcher, botanist, carpenter, needlepointer, mountain climber, and museum-goer, she has shown me that the world is an endlessly fascinating place—all of it worth learning and writing about. Her encouragement and editorial comments fueled me through the research and writing. She shall continue to inspire me all my life.

Three years ago, vaguely pondering the idea of this book, I attended a regional La Leche League (LLL) conference. After a morning of seminars, during which I realized that this conference was in every way like the professional seminars I had attended in the course of my career except that a multitude of babies and children were present, I arrived for the luncheon in the hotel ballroom. Looking around for an empty seat, and finding one at a table of strangers, I sat down next to Gerry Anne Dubis. An LLL leader from New Hampshire, Gerry Anne, as luck would have it, had helped countless working mothers to nurse their babies. By the time dessert was served, Gerry Anne and I were planning our own seminar to be given at the following LLL conference. Later she donated hours reviewing the text of the book and fixing inaccuracies; her experience and expertise are laced throughout these chapters. I am also grateful to Kittie Frantz, pediatric nurse-practitioner and professor of lactation at the University of Southern California Medical School, who provided a thoughtful review of the manuscript, invaluable expertise, and resources.

Kathleen Huggins, registered nurse and certified lactation consultant, and also the author of *The Nursing Mother's Companion* and co-author of *The Nursing Mother's Guide to Weaning*, came on deck as co-author for the second edition of this book. Her expertise in pumping and storing breast milk, as well as lactation management, ensure that *Nursing Mother, Working Mother* is as authoritative as it is supportive. Welcome aboard, Kathleen, and thank you. Meticulous editing by Linda Ziedrich and Dan Rosenberg also reassured me that this book would be the best it could be.

I owe special thanks, too, to the many mothers who corresponded with me across the Internet, sharing their concerns and solutions. Judith Ravel and the late Maurice (Reese) Wakeman, grandparents extraordinaire, kept my family in good company and well fed while I toiled. Reese taught me, as he did hundreds of parents in his pediatric practice, that all a parent really needs is confidence. Many others provided inspiration and practical help: Miranda Helin, Susan Polit, Mary Jane Daly, Deborah Sloan, Katharine MacPhail, Lisa May, Joanna Kolis, and still others—all shining examples of dedicated professionals who have kept their jobs from coming between their children and themselves—became my sounding boards over cups of tea and during walks in the woods. To them and the many others who have shared their lives and enthusiasm with me, I offer my thanks.

—G.P.

I WOULD LIKE TO THANK Gale Pryor for inviting me to assist her in this new edition of *Nursing Mother, Working Mother.* A special thanks to Linda Ziedrich for her more than two decades of guiding and editing my writing. I also wish to acknowledge, for their dedication to their breastfed children, the thousands of nursing-and-working mothers whom I have been involved with over the past twenty-five years. Of course, my writing has always been made possible by the love and support of my family, Brad, Kate, and John.

—K.H.

A note about the term *working mother*

*A*s anyone who has ever raised a child knows full well, all mothers are working mothers. Mothers with jobs heartily agree that the work they do at home is usually more physically exhausting and mentally taxing than the work they do for pay. Unfortunately, our language does not provide a useful and accurate term for those mothers who have major responsibilities outside the family as well as within it. The term *employed mothers* excludes both mothers who are employers and mothers who are students. *Working mothers* may seem to slight women without jobs, but it is all we are left with. Although written with the understanding that mothering requires as much effort and skill as any paid job, this book is about the challenge of combining dual social roles.

PREFACE

BY GALE PRYOR

"I am going back to work after the baby is born."

THE NECESSITY OF RETURNING TO WORK is one of the most common reasons that women decide against breastfeeding, or decide to wean after only a few weeks of nursing. And yet breastfeeding can be one of the best things a working mother ever does for herself or her baby.

In 1987, a few weeks before giving birth to my first child, I told my obstetrician that I planned to breastfeed even though I would be returning to work after an eight-week maternity leave. She said that I probably would be unable to pump enough milk to feed the baby during our separations, and that the baby probably wouldn't take a bottle, anyway. The day-care provider I'd chosen told me she didn't usually accept breastfed babies into her home because she didn't like keeping breast milk in her refrigerator. My boss turned pale and averted his eyes when I mentioned that I would need twenty minutes twice a day to pump my milk. He then denied me an extra, third month of maternity leave. Even my always supportive husband worried that I would be too exhausted to breastfeed while working.

Fortunately, about 30 years before, my mother, Karen Pryor, had breastfed my two brothers and me. She nursed us in a time when breastfeeding was an oddity, unfashionable and discouraged. She nursed despite being told that she couldn't breastfeed because all three of her children had been born by cesarean section (I still haven't figured out the reason for that). Rather than accepting those opinions and taking up the bottle, she got mad. She went to the library and read. She traveled to talk with other breastfeeding mothers. She learned all she could about breastfeeding, and she put it in a book, *Nursing Your Baby*, first published in 1963. Now in its fourth edition, her book has sold more than a million copies over 40 years, and it has helped mothers around the world joyfully nurse their babies.

Yet nearly 30 years after my mother bucked our culture's prejudice against breastfeeding, I was up against it in a new, subtler form. I began to see that, in our culture, the involved mothering that breastfeeding signifies was considered incompatible with a commitment to one's life in the working world. If I wanted to stay in a world in which success was modeled on men's lives, it was expected that I not also seek success in a traditionally feminine way. Make your choice, said our culture: children or career, mother or employee, woman or man. So I did what my mother did. I got mad.

I had just begun my career in a field that I loved, and I did not want to quit now. And I was determined to nurse my baby until he weaned himself. Eight weeks after my son Max was born, I returned to full-time work, pumping twice a day and nursing during the evenings, nights, and early mornings, and on the weekends. Max weaned at 18 months while I was away on a three-day business trip. I had proved my obstetrician and other naysayers wrong. Combining nursing and working wasn't impossible. Once I understood the schedule and the mechanics of pumping and storing milk, it wasn't even that hard. It wasn't breastfeeding that challenged me as a nursing, working mother.

I found that my new role as a mother continued to conflict with my life at work. I discovered that chatting about babies while waiting for a meeting to begin was considered unprofessional (whereas discussing the previous night's baseball game was not). My unwillingness to fly to Chicago at the drop of a hat was taken as evidence of a lack of commitment. I no longer stayed at work a minute past five o'clock, but rushed to the elevators and home to my baby, shrugging off thoughts of how my behavior was affecting my image as a hard worker. I split my life in two as I took on two incompatible identities. I felt terribly torn between excelling at the job I loved and learning this new, equally compelling job of motherhood.

Breastfeeding, however, far from becoming an additional source of stress, relieved my anxieties. My confidence suddenly shaken in arenas in which I once felt so sure, I knew that in this one function, nurturing my child, I was doing fine. Breastfeeding reassured me that even though Max spent much of the day with a babysitter he adored, I was irreplaceable to him. Only I could offer him a warm breast full of sweet milk. At the end of each day, when I nursed him before heading home from the sitter's house, there was no "getting to know you again" adjustment period. We were immediately a couple, instantly and completely in tune with one another.

There were myriad other benefits to Max and to me. Breastfeeding turned out to be more convenient than bottle feeding, a blessing considering my demanding schedule. Breastfeeding was relaxing, too. As soon as my milk let down, I found it difficult to remember what had vexed me so at the office that day, and I came to rely on the calm that always followed a peaceful nursing. Breastfeeding also helped me to focus on Max, and to make the most of my precious time with him. His fingers toying with the buttons on my blouse, his bright eyes looking up, and his quick smile that sent milk dribbling down his cheek as he nursed swept away worries about getting dinner made and laundry done. If I had bottle-fed Max, there would have been many a night when I might have propped him up with a bottle "just for a minute" while I put a pot on the stove or a load in the washing machine. Breastfeeding helped me remember that what my baby needed most of all was me.

Looking back, I realize that continuing to breastfeed while working tied the two halves of my life together and helped me make sense of myself as a mother. Breastfeeding gave my baby the best beginning, and also guided my first steps as his mother. The gentle, intuitive intimacy between a breastfed baby and his mother provided me with a blueprint for parenting my child long after weaning.

I found, too, that at work I could draw on the confidence I had acquired by successfully nursing my baby. I gained perspective on matters that once riled me. I began to extend to the world at large the calm acceptance, the warm receptivity that I had learned through breastfeeding.

Most importantly, however, continuing to breastfeed while working kept me from submerging the mother I had become beneath the working person I had long been. Breastfeeding helped me to become aware of, and then to resist, the pressure to pretend for eight hours a day that no baby was at home competing for, and balancing, my time and devotion. Breastfeeding was my declaration that I could get the job done as a woman rather than as a man.

Too often we bow to cultural pressure and accept the premise that employees do not have private lives, children do not have daily needs, and home and work are two separate spheres that never come in contact with each other. This living in two separate worlds at once, while obligated to meet the competing demands of each, is, I believe, the source of overwhelming stress for employed mothers. I hope that this book will help you combine your working life and your home life, through breastfeeding and sensitive parenting, to form a unity between yourself as a mother and the person you are on the job. I hope it will help you learn to blend both sides of your life, so that you may simultaneously raise your child, enjoy your work, and, perhaps, serve as an example to others that raising children is not a personal hobby, but a joyful responsibility that we must all take on together.

one

Bonding, Breastfeeding, and the Working Mother

*"I didn't expect to feel this way.
I can't take my eyes off my baby."*

B ECOMING A MOTHER is an experience full of surprises. The most astonishing surprise of all may be the intensity of your feelings for your new baby. Before your baby is born, you may have trouble imagining your life with a baby in it. After your baby is born, though, it may be difficult to imagine life without this new, extraordinary person. Becoming a mother is an experience that changes you forever.

The quality of the experience varies from woman to woman. For some, the first weeks and months of motherhood seem enchanted. For others, this is a period of transition and adjustment in which the enchantment of mothering occurs only gradually. In either case, the idea of returning to work outside the home after the baby is born may be unexpectedly hard to accept. Many pregnant women have never imagined how hard it would be to leave their babies.

How Mothers and Babies Bond

The first moments of motherhood have always fascinated observers of human behavior. In studying mothers and their newborns, researchers have identified a universal, elegant interplay that sparks the lifelong bond between mothers and their children.

A bond between any two people, including a mother and baby, develops and deepens over time. Babies, however, arrive in the world designed to initiate and establish that bond. Able to see, hear, smell, and feel with far more clarity than once assumed, newborns use their amazing innate abilities to make their parents want to care for them, want to help them grow and thrive. Your baby's first developmental task, one for which she has abundant talent, is to make you fall head over heels in love with her.

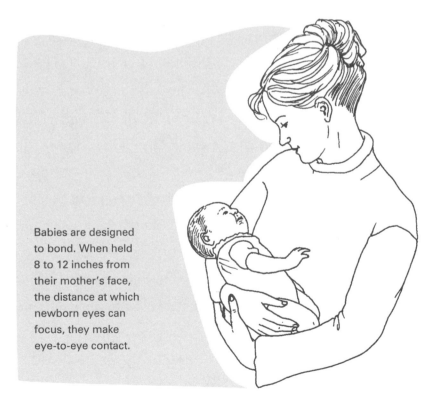

Babies are designed to bond. When held 8 to 12 inches from their mother's face, the distance at which newborn eyes can focus, they make eye-to-eye contact.

New mothers also behave in ways that seem to be instinctive. We almost always touch our newborns in the same way, first with our fingertips, then with the palms of our hands, moving from their extremities to their tummies and backs and lastly to their faces. We tend to hold our babies in what researchers call the *en face* position, so that our faces are 8 to 12 inches from our babies' faces, which happens to be the distance at which newborn eyes can most easily focus. We usually have an intense desire to make eye-to-eye contact with our babies, and we find their returned gaze immensely gratifying. We speak to our babies in high, soft voices reserved especially for them. And our babies employ myriad, enchanting ways that lead us to touch them, gaze at them, and speak to them ever more in a cycle of interactions that over time create a richly layered mother-child relationship.

John Kennell and Marshall Klaus, the pioneering researchers in mother-infant bonding, have described this intricate, instinctive pattern of interactions as "a fail-safe system that is over-determined to ensure the proximity of mother and child." The deep attachment arising from your natural interactions with your baby will allow you to meet his needs intuitively—and will help him to feel secure whenever he is close to you. Even if you and your newborn must be separated for a time just after birth—if one of you becomes ill, for example—your dance of attachment will continue, though at a slower tempo. And even if you are so overwhelmed with exhaustion, worry, or other feelings that falling in love must wait, you and your baby will, finally, become deeply bonded when you are ready. Once this happens, you will have formed the first strong strand of a lifelong bond that cannot easily be broken.

The Role of Breastfeeding in Bonding

Breastfeeding usually plays an integral role in forming the deep attachment between mother and baby. Bottle-feeding mothers, of course, also become securely attached to their babies. There are many tools in the attachment kit; breastfeeding is but one. It is, however, an extraordinarily powerful one.

Breastfeeding is designed by nature to over-ensure maternal-infant interaction and closeness. If done without schedules or other restrictions, breastfeeding guarantees that you and your baby will be in close physical contact 8 to 18 times in every 24 hours. In fact, nursing mothers tend to be with their infants altogether more than other mothers. In the first 10 days after birth, nursing mothers hold their babies more than bottle-feeding mothers do, even when they are not nursing. They rock their babies more, speak to their babies more, and are more likely to sleep with their babies. In Western society many women never hold a newborn until they give birth to their own, yet this frequent skin-to-skin contact and interaction soon make up for even a complete lack of familiarity with babies. The mother who immerses herself in her newborn, breastfeeding frequently and without restrictions, quickly learns to read her baby's cues and to trust her own instincts. She extends the gentle give-and-take, the empathy, and the commitment of breastfeeding into the rest of her mothering. Nursing her baby provides her with a blueprint for sensitive parenting in the years to come.

Nursing couples need each other physically and emotionally. The baby, of course, has a physical need for milk. As scientists have amply documented, breast milk benefits every system in a baby's body, in infancy and for a lifetime. Breastfeeding offers protection against allergies and respiratory infections, and perhaps obesity. It improves vision and oral development, reduces the incidence of ear infections, protects the cardiovascular system and kidneys, and enhances babies' intestinal immunity. Juvenile diabetes is less common among children who were breastfed than those who were bottle-fed. Heart disease and high blood pressure are less common among adults who were breastfed.

Breast milk is brain food. Breastfeeding enhances a baby's cognitive development partially because it allows the baby more control in feeding—and the ability to control one's own actions is essential in human development. And breast milk itself, with its high levels of the fatty acids DHA and AA, supports optimal brain development. Indeed, recent studies have found that children fed mother's milk as babies have higher IQs, on average, than those fed formula. In fact, the more breast milk consumed as an infant, the better a child's cognitive function. In a study published in 1999 in the *American Journal of Clinical Nutrition,* babies breastfed for at least the first six months had an average IQ five points higher than that of a bottle-fed control group. Other studies have shown as much as an eight-point increase.

Of course, a baby's emotional need for love and reassurance is just as strong as her physical need for milk. Whereas most formula-fed babies are soon taught to hold their own bottles, the breastfed baby is most often held by her mother for feedings. A breastfed baby enjoys not only the comfort of the warm breast, but caressing, rocking, and eye contact before, during, and after feedings. With all her senses, she drinks in her mother's love.

In the mutual nature of nursing, a mother has a physical need, too, for her baby to take the milk from her breasts. When your newborn begins to suck at your breast, or even just to mouth your nipple, the hormone oxytocin is released in your body, hastening the contraction of your uterus and inducing the let-down or milk-ejection reflex, which begins your milk flow. The let-down of milk is relieving, satisfying, like a drink of water when one is thirsty. Called "the love hormone" because it is also produced during sexual intercourse and birth, oxytocin brings on a sudden feeling of contentment and pleasure as you breastfeed your baby, and it increases your desire to hold and caress and respond to your baby. In this way, you and your baby become a happy team at feedings, each amply rewarded by the other for her efforts.

The Confident Parent

Successful breastfeeding not only tends to produce healthy, happy babies, it also creates confident mothers. Marianne Neifert, a pediatrician and mother of five, saw this in her practice. "I began to recognize the impact of early parenting experiences, such as breastfeeding, on long-term parental competency. A woman who received necessary support and information, which enabled her to breastfeed as long as she had planned, tended to look back on her experience with pride and satisfaction. Her confidence radiated to other areas of mothering, and she viewed herself as a competent and successful parent."

Large-scale research studies confirm Dr. Neifert's observations. In Colorado and Tennessee, researchers followed hundreds of families in which the mothers had received several visits from a maternal-child nurse or community educator in the first weeks after their babies were born. Breastfeeding support and other gentle teaching were offered at each visit. The benefits to both mothers and babies were dramatic and endured for years. Mothers who received visits, as opposed to a control group that did not, were more likely to begin and continue breastfeeding. They also reported less postpartum depression and more pleasure in mothering. Their children were observed up to six years later, and those who had been visited by a nurse and breastfed as babies demonstrated higher IQ and language scores and fewer behavioral problems than did children in the control group. The visited children also demonstrated better strategies for conflict resolution. Support for mothering had created confident mothering, which was more likely to include breastfeeding. That confidence shapes what we do and the people our children become.

> **"** Breastfeeding nudges other aspects of maternal behavior. **"**
>
> —NILES NEWTON

Breastfeeding's gift of confidence comes as you nurture your baby with your own body and mind. Parents who use formula may rely on manufacturers' and doctors' advice. Feeding our babies is the first and most fundamental responsibility of parenting. After that comes all else. If we develop little faith in our independent ability to perform that primary task, we may not be certain of our other abilities in the parenting still to come. Whereas a breastfeeding mother leaves milk composition, temperature, cleanliness, and intake up to her body and the baby's, for the formula-feeding parent these are all subjects for worry and debate, which may further erode her confidence.

Parenting styles differ enormously from family to family, and many different kinds of families produce happy, healthy children. Whatever their parenting style, though, mothers and fathers who are confident in themselves as parents tend to raise equally self-assured children. These parents not only teach self-esteem by modeling it, but because they are confident, say social researchers, they also tend to be empathetic rather than controlling. They respond reliably to their children's needs. Their children are more likely to feel secure, trusting, and confident in themselves and their environment.

Far more valuable than advice from relatives, friends, or experts is the knowledge *within* you that you are completely capable of caring for and raising your new baby. Bruno Bettelheim, the child psychologist, writes in *A Good Enough Parent* that "acting on the recommendations of others cannot evoke in us the feelings of confirmation that well up in us only when we have understood *on our own, in our own ways*, what is involved in a particular situation, and what we can therefore do about it." Successful breastfeeding seems, say experienced mothers, to kindle these "feelings of confirmation," for the breastfeeding mother knows in her heart that she can nurture her child well.

Breastfeeding, in short, is much more than a feeding method. Beyond providing perfect nutrition at every stage of your baby's growth, breastfeeding is a language, subtle and intimate, between you and your baby, as well as a proud and marvelous expression of your unique abilities as a woman and as a mother. It is a teacher when you are learning to trust your intuition as a mother, and it is a friend when you need the comfort of knowing you and your baby are indispensable to one another. When you return to work, breastfeeding will ensure that the bond between you and your baby cannot be weakened by your frequent separations.

The Risks of Working to Attachment

Falling in love and becoming in synch with our babies, a process called "attachment" in human development research, usually proceeds without our thinking about it much. We get pregnant, we give birth, we fall in love with our babies, we learn to breastfeed, we become mothers in tune with our babies. Voilà. We have accomplished one of life's major transitions, becoming a mother. Unless we don't.

Sometimes women don't fully traverse the divide between childless woman and mother. They have babies, but they resist the bone-deep commitment that comes with motherhood. After all, becoming a mother is a frightening, gigantic leap into a new and all-encompassing stage of life. Motherhood threatens to submerge both accomplishments of the past and goals for the future, as well as one's present sense of self. The fear of losing oneself in its floodwaters is entirely normal.

Besides, in American culture today, motherhood receives scant respect, especially among high-achievers. If your self-respect comes mainly from your success at work, especially if that work is competitive and pressured, reentering the world with *mother* suddenly attached to your identity can be dismaying, to say the least. Despite the impressive diplomatic and managerial skills that motherhood teaches women, the business world holds mothers in suspicion. We are widely suspected of not being truly committed to our jobs and our employers—and any child-related activity that intrudes upon our work simply confirms that suspicion.

Katharine Ellison, in her book *The Mommy Brain: How Motherhood Makes Us Smarter*, cites Princeton University researchers who conducted an opinion poll about working mothers. They found clear evidence of this shift in attitude toward employed women returning from maternity leaves. "When working women become mothers," writes Ellison, "they unwittingly make a trade—perceived warmth for perceived competence. This trade unjustly costs them professional credibility and hinders their odds of being hired, promoted, and generally supported in the workplace." Men, on the other hand, are more likely to reap professional benefits as they receive, with the advent of fatherhood, what Ellison calls, "the cachet of stability."

Women first broke into predominantly male fields of work by disproving feminine stereotypes and by proving that they could do the work as well, *and in the same way,* as men. In the 1970s and 1980s, women edging into the corporate world wore outfits that replicated men's business suits except that the bottom half ended in one hem rather than two. They often avoided having traditionally feminine hobbies and traits. They strived to prove they could be at least as tough, and work at least as long, as any man. Entry into the world of men required *being,* as much as possible, like men. If women wanted equal opportunities, they had to adhere to the existing norms of the workplace.

No doubt becoming mock men was a necessary step in the effort to open doors for women. Many women who now hold high positions in U.S. corporations or in the professions forfeited having children. As Sylvia Ann Hewlett writes in *Creating a Life: Professional Women and the Quest for Children,* "these highly accomplished women vaulted over barriers and crashed through glass ceilings, but found it extraordinarily difficult—if not impossible—to have children as well." Women who did manage to have children along the way found that their professional lives required them to behave as if their children did not exist.

In many regions and industries, this requirement remains. One attorney just back from a three-month maternity leave says, "I'm working very hard to reestablish myself as a lawyer, not a mommy. It's gotten to the point where I almost refuse to talk about the baby in the office." *Breaking the Glass Ceiling,* a report on executive women published in 1992, advised, "For women, it is more important that they visibly limit their family life and personal relationships to convince others that they are committed. . . . The obvious solution for women who want to demonstrate their commitment to the corporation and thereby earn a chance for advancement into the executive suite is to give up everything else, including a family." More than a decade later, Hewlett writes, "the tough trade-offs faced by middle-aged women dog the footsteps of today's younger women. Indeed, women between the ages of 28 and 40 seem to be having an even harder time balancing career and children than their older sisters." We're still working on this old problem. Cornell University researchers recently found that employers still tend to perceive working mothers as less competent, committed, and deserving of promotion than childless women who are equally qualified. In their study, published in 2005, applicants whose resumés indicated that they were mothers were hired half as frequently and, if hired, offered an average $11,000 less in starting pay. Employers, reported the researchers, "expect mothers are going to be less committed to their jobs."

Without diminishing those brave and determined women who broke new ground for all of us, it would be a bizarre and backward success story if feminism's final chapter were about women becoming, for all intents and purposes, men. Surely feminism's triumph will come when women can work in any field they choose without having to sacrifice the joys and commitment of motherhood. Will not our society be a better one when mothers can openly nurture their children without risking their careers—when we are able to embrace motherhood without apology? Certainly the lives of children will be improved.

The result of our social revolution is that new mothers returning to their working worlds confront a culture that still doesn't quite know what to do with them. Beyond requests for maternity leaves and flexible hours, there lies another barrier. The general confusion in our culture about roles of women and images of accomplishment compounds the very personal challenge of changing from working woman into working mother. Flummoxed by the cultural confusion, a woman may resist the transition altogether, circumventing the conflict between work and motherhood by continuing to live her life as if having a baby has had little if any impact on it. Unfortunately, in the process, a distance, an unfamiliarity and mutual discomfort, may come between her and her baby.

This distancing may begin in the hospital. A new mother may choose to bottle-feed because she believes that her return to work will require her to wean within a few weeks in any case. She may believe that formula is just as healthy for her baby as breast milk, and a lot more convenient for her. She may have been told that once she starts breastfeeding, she will never get the baby to take a bottle. She may even believe that returning to work will be easier for both her and her baby if she does not allow her baby to become completely dependent on her now. If she wants to try breastfeeding, she might ask the nurses to teach her to use a breast pump even before her milk comes in, for she is focusing on the day she'll return to work. She may end up feeding her baby pumped breast milk, and rarely if ever putting the baby to the breast.

A new mother already mentally preparing for her return to work may accept the nurses' advice (still all too common) to leave her baby in the nursery except at feeding times so that she herself can get some rest. Allowing the maternity ward staff to care for her newborn, she may leave the hospital with the sense that she barely knows her baby.

At home, she begins caring for her baby in ways she hopes will promote independence. She hopes to have her baby sleeping through the night before her first day back at work, even if this means letting him "cry it out." Her primary goal during her maternity leave is to hire a satisfactory babysitter or to find an opening in a daycare home or center. She may even hire a professional baby nurse to help out until she can find a long-term caregiver. She may take advice like that offered by a guide for career women written in the 1980s, which encourages mothers to "make the most of their maternity leaves" by "calling the office at 10:00 A.M. and 4:00 P.M. every day and going to the office once a week for key meetings." In short, she focuses on the management job of combining motherhood with her working life, rather than on becoming her baby's mother.

When her maternity leave is over and this mother is back at work, the hours there seem comfortingly familiar, unlike the time she spends with the little stranger at home. At work the mother's activities are well organized. She can begin and complete a task without interruption. Her work has tangible results. She chats with adults about anything other than her baby because she feels she must reestablish her professional image. Pictures of her baby are limited to a discreet frame on her desk.

If she is still breastfeeding at all, this mother may give pumping a try, but she quickly finds that she doesn't get much milk with the pump she picked up at the pharmacy. Her milk seems to be drying up anyway, and her baby really does seem to prefer the bottle. She soon gives up the idea of pumping and, shortly afterward, of nursing as well. She may be relieved or she may feel a bit blue about this, but everyone (her doctor, other working mothers, and her relatives) has told her that this would probably happen.

At home, the skills that make her a star at work seem no help in her role as a parent. She grows increasingly dependent on child-care advice from the babysitter, and she begins to feel that perhaps she is just not temperamentally suited to this mothering business. Perhaps, she thinks, it's better to delegate her child's care to trained professionals. As one mother declares, "I do not regret working, and here's why: One, I am providing my son with a role model, showing that adults need to work and that women work as well as men; and two, I am not a 'professional' child rearer, and I want only the best for my baby." Although this mother surely loves her baby as deeply as any other parent does, she does not trust or respect herself as a mother. The admiration she receives from her coworkers and the rest of society—for joining the ranks of those amazing superwomen, able to "do it all" without a hair out of place—confirms her decision to delegate child rearing.

Unseen is the distance that may be developing between her and her baby. For the mother who lacks confidence in her own abilities to nurture her baby, this distance enables her life to proceed more or less as though a child had never entered the picture. Her baby is growing and developing as he is designed to do, but she is not developing as his mother. She finds it hard to understand why he cries and how to calm him. As he becomes a toddler, they may lock horns frequently as she searches for solutions from friends and experts to the problem of raising her "difficult" child. She and her child love each other deeply, but they are not in harmony.

The risk in returning to work after a baby is born is not that a mother and baby will be apart for many hours, but that working increases the chance that their lives will run on separate tracks, at different speeds, and in opposite directions. Working, especially at a job that demands that a woman display her commitment daily, can lead her to live two concurrent, incompatible lives. The risk is not created by the hours away from the baby, but by the expectations of the place in which she works.

To prove her commitment to her job, too often a woman must obscure her life as a mother. She may soon find herself living two separate lives, switching from one role to another each day. The competing commitments of work and motherhood may eventually cause one to dominate the other. For many women, life with a baby wins. Some continue paid employment but stop giving their hearts and souls to their jobs. Those who have the option may continue to work a reduced schedule or with less responsibility, or may even stop altogether for a few years. For other women work life dominates, and being a mother may ebb to second place. A fortunate few find a way to blend their roles into one identity that travels to meet the needs of both commitments. The women who achieve that fluidity seem to share an unwillingness to apologize for either part of their lives.

Child-development specialists have expressed concern about the impact of work in which a woman must prove her commitment at the expense of motherhood. As Dr. Michael Bulmash, a clinical psychologist in Stamford, Connecticut, contends, we have "created a generation of mothers who are losing the ability to pick up on cues and signals from their children." While in every generation there are mothers who read their children well and mothers who do not, the concern that social and economic pressures may distance us from our children is well founded.

Research on working mothers and their attachment to their children has produced mountains of conflicting and subtle data. We do know, however, that working outside the home lessens the likelihood of breastfeeding. A study from the Bendheim Thoman Center for Research on Child Wellbeing at Princeton University found that mothers who expect to work in the year following the birth of their child have 15 percent lower odds of breastfeeding than other mothers. They also found that mothers who plan to work after the child is born may not initiate breastfeeding at all because of the anticipated difficulties in combining breastfeeding and employment. The working mothers in the study had 48 percent higher odds of weaning within one month after returning to work, and 46 percent higher odds in the month preceding a return to work, as compared with mothers who were not getting ready to work. If breastfeeding is a mother's first teacher in reading her child's cues and signals, the loss of the nursing relationship because of the pressures of work ripples far and wide.

Once we are aware of societal pressure to surrender or minimize motherhood, however, it can be resisted. You *can* stay close to your baby, despite the demands of your job, by finding ways, such as breastfeeding, that will help you to feel confident in your mothering skills, to know your baby's unique cues and character, and to develop as a mother alongside your developing baby.

> Working outside your home does not mean that you will inevitably be less in tune with your baby than an at-home mother. With awareness and understanding, you can erase the risk of this happening.

To minimize the risk of distancing between mothers and babies, we must change our culture's views of working and mothering. The lack of support for parenting in general, and its grievous consequences, has been well documented by writers and researchers, among them Sylvia Ann Hewlett and Cornel West in their 1998 book, *The War Against Parents*. The gap between idealized motherhood and support for the real work of mothering is especially wide for employed women. Gunn Johansson, a professor of work psychology at the University of Stockholm, compared the lives of female managers in Sweden and the former West Germany. Although the two societies are similar in many ways, Sweden provides a broader range of benefits, including extended maternity leaves and high-quality child care, to all its families. In Sweden, the study revealed, most of the female managers have at least two children; in Germany, most are single women with no children. German women feel they must forsake family for work, Johansson concludes, whereas Swedish women consider it their right to combine the two roles. In Sweden, the needs of mothering are recognized by the culture at large and real support is provided to meet them.

Here in the United States, working women's benefits depend on the goodwill of private corporations rather than federal policy. If employers offer benefits in response to the real needs of working parents, employees have a greater chance of succeeding as both workers and parents. Short, unpaid maternity leaves, long working hours, inflexible schedules, and scant health benefits are well-recognized impediments to combining work and family. While in some industries enlightened policies for families are on the rise, the additional pressure on American women to further their careers by minimizing motherhood is still a common aspect of corporate culture. How easily you combine mothering and work, therefore, may depend on the type of work you do, the region in which you do it, and for whom.

Working Mothers through History

So what are we to do? Devote our lives to fulfilling careers at the expense of harmonious relationships with our children? Give up our jobs to be perfect mothers and raise perfect children?

Women who choose the latter course sometimes think they're assuming a traditional role. But the truth is that mothers have always worked. In hunting, foraging, and agricultural societies, women's work—and not just nurturing—has through the millennia been indis-

pensable to the survival of their families and communities. In most
of the world today, this remains true. Outside of the highly industrialized countries, 90 percent of women must work for their and their
families' living. Forty percent of the world's farmers are women.
Where are their children while they work? Their babies ride on their
backs or nestle against their bosoms in slings, while their older children toddle nearby or help out as best they can. A mother pauses in
her work to nurse, and then returns to it while her child plays beside
her or naps against her body, lulled by her motions. Or a grandmother
or other relative watches over a group of children as their mothers
work. As the children grow, they pitch in, having seen the work that
must be done and how it must be done. Irenaus Eibl-Eibesfeldt, an
ethologist who has studied tribal societies across the globe, points
out that in most of these societies, women spend at least 40 hours a
week working—and working hard. These mothers would be most surprised to hear that being economically productive and being the
mother of small children should be mutually exclusive.

In the West, too, through most of history, it would have been in-
conceivable for the great majority of women not to combine child
care with work. Women's gardens, looms, and livestock formed the
basis of cottage industry until the middle of the nineteenth century.
A fascinating account of laboring women (in both senses of the word)
is found in *The Midwife's Tale: The Life of Martha Ballard, Based on
Her Diary 1785-1812,* by Laurel Thatcher Ulrich. Martha Ballard was
a mother of nine and the midwife for 816 babies of other women who
lived in and around Hallowell, Maine. Her diary documents how Early
American women, like women before them, made their livings as they
raised their children. Martha and other women in her community
kept their own accounting books, documenting their trade in goods
and services. Medicine, textiles, and garden produce were "strands of
a broad and largely invisible local economy managed by women,"
writes Ulrich. These women, cultivating and preserving so that one
harvest season stretched almost to the next, certainly worked as hard
as we do. Their work, however, unlike that of many women today, did

not require them to be separated from their children or to submerge their identities as mothers. Traditional women's work blended well with the raising of children.

The Industrial Revolution at first changed only the location of women's work. When industry moved from the cottage to the factory, both women and children moved along with it. This change in venue was disastrous for children, of course, who worked in exhausting, often dangerous jobs until child-labor laws were enacted in the early twentieth century. Eventually most factories become the province of a male work force, while most women remained at home, raising children, gardening, cooking, and sewing. These domestic crafts, however, gradually lost their economic necessity and clout; they were and are relegated to the trivial status of hobbies. During World War II most American women took jobs, to replace the men who had enlisted, but the women were ousted at the end of the war to make way for returning soldiers. It was only then, in the late 1940s and 1950s, that the role of women as exclusively wives and mothers became a cultural ideal.

Of course, retiring to raise children was and is possible only for women whose husbands earn enough money to support a family. In economically disadvantaged and single-parent families, women have never had the choice to be full-time at-home mothers. These women have always blended work and family, apologizing for neither, providing for both as best they could.

The period in which mothers were supposed to be economically unproductive to dedicate themselves to full-time child care and housework was but a brief blip in Western history. Today that period is over; more than 60 percent of U.S. mothers of children under one year of age work outside their homes. In fact, the image of the "traditional family"—a working father, a homemaking mother, and one or more children—now represents only 9 percent of U.S. households. Nevertheless, the full-time homemaker lives on as a cultural ideal, spreading guilt among women who cannot live up to both her image and that of the career woman.

Mothers are working again. What is new is that we must be separated from our children while we work. And when we enter traditionally male fields, not only are we physically separated for most of each day, but we find we must be emotionally separated from our children as well.

What's Next?

Families today are reeling from the effects of these fundamental shifts in the structure of our lives. After all, as a species we have spent one hundred thousand years evolving physically, socially, and instinctually. In the tiniest final fraction in the time line of our existence, we've rearranged nearly all of our social structures and denied much of our well-honed instinctual knowledge. We attempt even to fight our physical evolution as we go to extremes in exercising and dieting, and hold up bizarre physical attributes as cultural standards of beauty. We are rethinking, reshaping who we are as human beings. We've thrown the entire deck of cards into the air and they are raining down in disarray upon the heads of parents and children, who together make up the single social unit that has remained a constant since the beginning of human existence.

How then do we pick ourselves up, dust off the cultural flotsam and jetsam, and find the methods both new and old that are truly helpful to us as we give birth to babies, raise children, and perform useful, satisfying work? This book is an exploration of a few methods of combining work and parenting that have worked for others now and in the past—beginning with breastfeeding, the most time honored, efficient, successful method of nurturing our babies while getting on with our lives.

two

WHY BREASTFEEDING IS IMPORTANT FOR YOU AND YOUR BABY

"Does it really matter whether I breastfeed my baby or not?"

D ESPITE THE INDISPUTABLE EVIDENCE, the debate continues. Does it really make a difference whether a baby is breastfed or bottle-fed? The answer is yes. No less of an authority than the American Academy of Pediatrics declares, in a 2005 policy statement on breastfeeding: "Extensive research, especially in recent years, documents diverse and compelling advantages to infants, mothers, families, and society from breastfeeding and the use of human milk for infant feeding. These include health, nutritional, immunologic, developmental, psychological, social, economic, and environmental benefits."

Although there are many reasons to choose to breastfeed your baby, perhaps the most compelling is that breast milk is filled with elements that provide optimum nourishment for your baby and protect her health in dozens of ways, now and far into the future. Some of these elements have yet to be identified, and many cannot be replicated by formula manufacturers now or ever.

In the past, scientists assumed that the reason breastfed babies had fewer infections than formula-fed babies was that breastfeeding allows less opportunity for contamination than bottle feeding does. Whereas milk taken directly from the breast has no chance to be contaminated, formula, which is mixed with water, put in a bottle, drunk through an artificial nipple, and perhaps left out and drunk again later, has repeated opportunities to grow bacteria. But even infants fed rigorously sterilized formula have higher rates of meningitis, diarrhea, and ear, respiratory, and urinary tract infections than breast-fed babies do. Scientists searched for another explanation why bottle-fed babies tend to be sick more often.

Laboratory investigations have since produced volumes of proof that breast milk defends babies against infection, besides having myriad other health benefits. Many of the investigating scientists, in fact, have turned into dedicated lactophiles with an abiding fascination for human milk. With every new discovery, their respect grows for the elegant efficiency of nature's system for nurturing babies. And working mothers who pump their breast milk on their lunch hours in borrowed offices and parked cars are doing so because they, too, understand that their own milk has no equal.

The Immunologic Benefits of Breast Milk

All mammals feed their babies with milk. But just as a mouse differs from a whale, a cat from a kangaroo, and a woman from a cow, each species' milk differs from that of other species. Horses and cows produce milk that grows bone and muscle quickly for babies that must be able to stand, walk, and run from the day of their birth. The very high-fat milk of a whale enables its baby to double its size in a few weeks and to withstand the cold seas. The milk of primates, including humans, promotes the rapid growth of brain tissue.

Infant mammals can survive on the milk of other species. Pigs have nursed kittens, and cats have nursed piglets. But young mammals fed this way miss out on the milk that is uniquely and perfectly designed for their own optimal growth and development. This is especially true if the species are very different, as are humans and cows.

> **"**The problems are great when you must modify the milk of hooved animals for infant human beings—if you wanted a really good match for us, you'd have to milk gorillas.**"**
>
> —KAREN PRYOR, *NURSING YOUR BABY, 4TH ED.*

So what is our own, perfectly tailored breast milk made of? To begin with, human milk is alive; fresh from the breast, it contains one million living cells per milliliter (or about one-third of a teaspoon). Colostrum, the honey-colored fluid that nourishes your baby for the first few days of life, contains up to seven million living cells per milliliter. Your placenta and blood nourished and protected your baby before birth, and your breasts, colostrum, and breast milk are designed to carry on the same vital functions after birth.

Most of the living cells in human milk are white cells similar to those in our blood. White cells search out and attack foreign bacteria on the surface of the baby's digestive organs and in the baby's tissues. Colostrum, the first milk, is full of white blood cells, so right from the beginning your newborn is protected against Coxsackie B virus and the bacteria *Salmonella,* streptococci, pneumococci, and the particularly nasty *E. (Escherichia) coli.* Every swallow your baby takes of colostrum or breast milk contains a tiny army of leukocytes and macrophages that surrounds and destroys the germs in its path. Although peak production of these protective cells occurs right after birth, they continue to be produced in effective quantities throughout the first year of nursing. In fact, levels of lysozyme, an enzyme produced by white cells that dissolves the cell walls of pathogens and is present in breast milk in quantities five thousand times higher than in cow's milk, actually increase for six months after birth and remain high through at least the second year of lactation.

Thanks to this battalion of anti-infective cells, human milk is a far more stable substance than pasteurized cow's milk or formula. If a container of breast milk is left open in a warm room for several hours, it is likely to have a *lower* bacteria count hours later than it did at first. The protective forces in breast milk will have spent those hours scouring the milk for pathogens and destroying them. The white cells in breast milk can even survive freezing if the milk has been properly stored, and they proceed with their work when the milk is thawed. But they cannot survive heating, including microwaving and pasteurization. And they cannot be created artificially.

Human breast milk is also teeming with protective immunoglobulins. There are five basic types of immunoglobulins, and all are present in human milk. The most abundant type is known as secretory IgA. Produced in your breasts, IgA molecules bind themselves to pathogens that may find their way into your baby's stomach and intestines, and thereby prevent them from entering the tissues lining the gastrointestinal tract. In the early months, your baby's intestines are highly permeable, allowing proteins and other foreign molecules to pass through and into your baby's blood. IgA coats these vulnerable surfaces, forming a protective shield against infections and allergens. Babies begin to produce secretory IgA on their own six to nine months after birth, but until then breast milk is their only source of this extraordinary protection.

Secretory IgA also enhances the effectiveness of the antibodies your body produces and passes through your milk to your baby. Your collection of antibodies matches the pathogens found in your and your nursing baby's environment. Whenever you ingest, inhale, or otherwise come in contact with a pathogen, your immune system manufactures an antibody designed to fight that specific germ. The constellation of antibodies that you pass on to your baby through your milk protects her from those same pathogens, the ones that your baby is most likely to encounter. Unfortunately, antibodies can cause inflammation as they surround and attack disease-causing organisms, and inflammation may scar delicate lung and intestinal tissues. Secretory IgA molecules enable antibodies to ward off infection without causing damaging inflammation.

Yet more components of breast milk add to the arsenal of anti-infectives that keep your baby safe. The Bifidus factor promotes the growth of a beneficial organism, *Lactobacillus bifidus,* that crowds out harmful organisms in the gut. This benign intestinal flora is the reason breastfed babies' stools lack the strong smell of formula-fed babies'. Lactoferrin, a protein not found in cow's milk, limits the growth of bacteria, especially *Staphylococcus aureus,* by binding to the iron they thrive on and disrupting their digestion of carbohydrates. Similarly, the B_{12}-binding protein inhibits the spread of bacteria by depriving them of the vitamin B_{12}. Interferon, present in mature milk and in teeming quantities in colostrum, is a well-known antiviral agent. Fatty acids found in breast milk damage the membranes of certain viruses, including the one that causes chicken pox, and may protect babies against intestinal parasites such as *Giardia lamblia* and *Entamoeba histolytica,* which causes amoebic dysentery. Fibronectin, a protein in breast milk, enhances the ability of white cells to hunt for pathogens. This protein, like secretory IgA, helps to minimize inflammation; indeed, fibronectin may actually help repair tissue that has been damaged by inflammation. According to recent studies, numerous hormones and proteins in colostrum and breast milk cause the immune systems of breastfed babies to mature sooner than those of formula-fed babies. Probably for this reason, breastfed babies produce higher levels of antibodies in response to immunizations than do formula-fed babies.

Scientists continue to be intrigued by the powers of human breast milk, and to explore its significance to lifelong health. More discoveries are sure to come. Already clear, however, is that breast milk provides babies with far more than nutrients. In diverse and remarkable ways, breastfeeding protects your baby until his own immune system begins to function independently, and far into the future.

The Nutritive Value of Breast Milk

Of course, the fundamental purpose of breast milk is to nourish your baby—and the ways in which it does so are just as impressive as the ways in which it protects your baby from disease. Human milk is a solution of protein, sugar, and salts in which a variety of fatty compounds are suspended. This milk provides all the necessary nutrients and fluid for babies from birth to six months of age, and guarantees that older babies have a constant, easily digestible source of essential vitamins, protein, carbohydrates, cholesterol, and trace elements while they are beginning to eat solid foods.

Unlike formula out of a can, mother's milk varies from one woman to another, from one week to the next, and even from hour to hour through the day. Its changes seem to correspond to the growing baby's changes in appetite and nutritional needs. The milk produced by mothers of premature babies, for example, is much higher in protein than that of mothers of full-term babies.

Fat provides 40 to 50 percent of the calories in breast milk. Despite many adults' dedicated avoidance of it, fat is essential for babies; it provides the energy they need to accomplish their astonishing growth rate. The fat in breast milk includes triglycerides, which are especially easy to digest, and prostaglandins. Although their function is not fully understood, prostaglandins may affect many physiologic processes, including circulation, gastric and mucous secretion, electrolyte balance, and zinc absorption.

The amount of fat in human milk varies according to several factors. Milk gets creamier over the course of a feeding, so the milk a baby gets at the end of the feeding is richest in fat. Also, the fat content of human milk goes up and down throughout the day, and is generally highest in the midmorning or early afternoon. Working mothers who pump their milk at these times provide their babies with especially hearty meals for the following day.

Recent research has focused on the role of fat in breast milk in brain development, in particular the fatty acids DHA and AA.

Although numerous studies have shown that children who were breastfed generally have IQs five to eight points higher at the age of eight than children who were formula-fed, the difference, some argued, could be attributed to environmental factors. Western mothers who choose to breastfeed their babies are more likely to be well educated, the argument went, and this may translate to higher IQs for their children. Breastfeeding hormones promote holding and cuddling, and physical interaction between a mother and her baby also promotes a baby's cognitive development.

But the claim that environmental rather than dietary factors led to higher IQ scores in breastfed children was refuted by studies in which premature babies were fed breast milk by bottle. Although they were never fed directly from the breast, these children scored higher on IQ tests years later than a control group of preemies who had been fed only formula.

New studies have pinpointed a nutritional cause of the statistically higher IQs of breastfed children. One study found significant differences in cognitive development (memory, problem solving, language) and visual development between babies fed formulas containing DHA and AA (derived from algae rather than breast milk) and babies fed formulas without these fatty acids. Studies of breastfed babies and formula-fed babies, even formulas with added synthetic DHA and AA, show the same difference. The breastfed babies have improved cognitive and visual function over even babies fed enriched formulas.

Studies that have considered the duration of breastfeeding show that the longer children are breastfed, the greater their IQ scores and school performance in the years ahead. Of course, after all the data crunching, it's just common sense: The human brain grows most rapidly during the first two years of life. Breast milk supports this growth, just as it does every other aspect of infant development.

Babies need cholesterol, too, and breast milk provides it in the appropriate quantity. In fact, cholesterol levels in human milk are quite high, whereas they are low in cow's milk and present in only trace quantities in formula. Cholesterol is required by your baby's rapidly growing nervous system. Although breastfed babies tend to have higher-than-average cholesterol levels as infants, when these babies reach adolescence and adulthood their cholesterol levels tend to be lower than average. Several studies of teenagers and adults suggest that breastfeeding may promote lifelong low cholesterol levels and a healthy cardiovascular system.

The principal sugar in human milk is lactose, and it is present in far greater quantity in human milk than in other animal milks. Human milk contains 20 to 30 percent more lactose than cow's milk does, which is why human milk tastes so much sweeter. Lactose promotes the growth of beneficial bacteria in your baby's intestines, inhibits the growth of harmful bacteria, and enhances numerous other protective functions. Lactose enhances calcium absorption, so important to your baby's growing bones, and breaks down to produce galactose, an essential nutrient for the development of brain tissue. In fact, researchers have observed that, among all mammals, the more lactose found in the milk, the larger the brain of the species. Since human milk contains so much more lactose than do formulas derived from cow's milk, the myriad benefits of lactose are more available to the breastfed than the bottle-fed infant.

Different animals grow at different rates, and these rates are apparently related to the level of protein in each species' milk. Humans grow more slowly than any other mammal, and human milk contains the least protein. Calves grow quite quickly, and cow's milk (and formula derived from it) is high in protein. The major proteins found in human and cow's milk are casein and whey, but, whereas cow's milk contains 80 percent casein and 20 percent whey, whey predominates in human milk. With its low casein content, human milk in the stomach forms small, soft, almost liquid curds that are easily digested, supplying a continuous flow of nutrients to the baby. In contrast, cow's milk, with its high casein content, forms a tough, rubbery curd that requires a high expenditure of energy for an incomplete digestion. The outdated recommendation that all babies, breastfed or bottle-fed, be fed at four-hour intervals is based on the amount of time it takes a baby to digest the large curds of cow's milk. The idea that a baby will sleep longer if given a bottle of formula also stems from this longer, more difficult, and less effective digestive process. The stomach of the breastfed baby empties rapidly and easily, while the baby absorbs nearly all the nutrients provided by the milk. Consequently, the baby wants to nurse more often, generally every hour and a half to three hours, for the first two to three months after birth. This in turn stimulates the mother's milk production and establishes her milk supply.

The human infant uses the protein in breast milk with nearly 100 percent efficiency. Virtually all the protein in breast milk becomes part of the baby; little or none is excreted. The baby fed on cow's milk-based or vegetable-based formula, however, may waste about half the protein in his diet. Some of the protein passes undigested through his system and is excreted in the feces. Some that is digested cannot be utilized by the cells of the body, and so is excreted in the urine. To get enough usable protein, the bottle-fed baby must drink a much larger volume of liquid than the breastfed baby. A working mother who knows this isn't concerned when her baby drinks one 8-ounce bottle of pumped breast milk at daycare for another baby's two or three bottles of formula.

Cystine, another protein not found in formula but abundant in human milk, is essential to skeletal growth. Although the blood of breastfed infants is rich in cystine, that of infants fed formula contains much less of this important protein.

One of the most striking differences between human and cow's milk lies in their mineral composition. This difference, like that in protein levels, may be related to the rate of growth of the species for which the milk was intended. Human milk contains less than a quarter as much calcium as cow's milk; this appears to be all the calcium a full-term baby needs. In the first year of life, babies on cow's milk-based diets grow larger and heavier skeletons than breastfed babies. Until recently, infant growth charts were based on the growth patterns of formula-fed babies. These charts have for decades misled pediatricians and parents into believing that big bones and the overall growth pattern of these babies is optimal. Exclusively breastfed babies tend to grow more quickly than formula-fed babies but are somewhat leaner, and their rate of growth tends to slow down at six months of age. New growth charts reflect this difference, and may reassure parents that their breastfed babies' growth is just as it should be.

Iron, needed to make red blood cells, was once thought to be absent from breast milk. Now known to be present in low levels, the iron in breast milk has a high "bioavailability"; nearly 50 percent of it is absorbed by the baby's body. In contrast, only 10 percent of iron in plain cow's milk and 4 percent of iron in iron-fortified infant formulas is absorbed; the rest is digested or excreted through the kidneys.

There are other micronutrients in human milk whose roles are not yet completely understood. Until a baby's need for a trace element is proven, formula manufacturers will not add it to their mixes. Infant formula, therefore, may lack many important micronutrients. Breast milk provides your baby with all necessary nutrients, whether or not scientists understand their significance.

Another significant difference between breastfeeding and formula feeding is that breastfeeding provides absolutely fresh milk, with all its vitamins still present. In the manufacture, storage, and reheating of formula, some vitamins are inevitably lost. Of course, some nutrients are lost when breast milk is frozen for long periods or reheated. Breast milk, however, is remarkably stable, much more so than formula or pasteurized cow's milk, and keeps most of its essential qualities through chilling, freezing, and heating.

As long as a breastfeeding mother eats a variety of nourishing foods and gets 15 minutes of sunshine on most days to ensure that her body manufactures sufficient vitamin D (30 minutes may be needed if a mother has a dark complexion), she can be assured that her milk will satisfy the vitamin and mineral requirements of a full-term, healthy baby. Even when the mother's diet is not ideal, breast milk supplies all the nutrients babies need for their first five to six months. And breast milk continues to be a good source of nutrients later, as a baby begins to eat solid foods. Mothers who breastfeed into the second and third year take comfort that their toddlers, so often picky eaters, are still receiving the spectrum of nutrients they need with each nursing.

Breast Milk and Allergies

Food allergies are believed to begin when foreign molecules penetrate the walls of a baby's intestinal tract and enter the bloodstream, causing mild to life-threatening reactions. Because the breastfed baby has received the benefit of secretory IgA and other elements that soothe and seal his intestinal surfaces, the baby can digest foreign proteins and molecules instead of absorbing them into his bloodstream. The formula-fed infant, however, may absorb whole proteins, and develop allergic reactions to them, well into her second year.

Allergic reactions are far less common in breastfed than in formula-fed babies. Cow's milk, eggs, chocolate, or citrus fruit in a mother's diet occasionally causes colic, or severe crying spells, in her breastfed baby, and if the mother drinks more than a few cups of coffee in a day, her baby may get jittery. Babies often outgrow sensitivities to any foods to which they may be exposed through their mothers' milk. In the meantime, their symptoms are quickly relieved when the mother stops eating the offending food. (Peanuts and tree nuts seem to be an exception. The increasing prevalence of peanut allergies and other nut allergies among children has led researchers to recommend that pregnant and nursing mothers avoid these foods to reduce their infants' exposure and the risk of developing an allergy.) Formula-fed babies experiencing allergic reactions to proteins in cow's milk or soy formula may not find relief so easily. Many are allergic to all but the very expensive hypoallergenic, or "predigested," formulas.

By six months of age, when nature intends a baby to sample new foods, food allergies are much less likely to become established. At this point many working mothers put away their pumps and allow their babies to be given formula or solids during their separations. Babies born into families with allergies, however, tend to begin producing secretory IgA later than do babies from families without this genetic inheritance. So if you have a family history of food allergies, you may want to delay the introduction of foods other than breast milk, especially those to which family members are allergic.

How do the immunologic and nutritive properties of human milk actually affect a baby's health? As study after study shows, exclusively breastfed babies have lower rates of diarrhea, vomiting, gastrointestinal infections, respiratory infections, and eczema than formula-fed babies do. Breastfed babies have less chance of succumbing to Sudden Infant Death Syndrome (SIDS). *Pediatrics*, the journal of the American Academy of Pediatrics, reported in 2004 that, in the United States, "children who were breastfed had a much lower risk of dying in the postneonatal period than infants never breastfed. Additionally, the longer the infants were breastfed, the lower the risk of postneonatal death." In 2006, *Pediatrics* published another study confirming that early and exclusive breastfeeding can make "a major contribution" to infant health worldwide. The report concluded that "16 percent of neonatal deaths could be saved if all infants were breastfed from day one and 22 percent if breastfeeding started within the first hour."

Breast milk's benefits continue long after weaning. As numerous studies have shown, children who were fed breast milk tend to score better on measures of cognitive function (language, math, memory, and problem solving) than their formula-fed peers. Babies who are exclusively breastfed for at least six months, likewise, have less chance of developing childhood cancer, juvenile rheumatoid arthritis, or juvenile diabetes. They also appear less likely to develop multiple sclerosis, Crohn's disease, celiac disease, Type 2 diabetes, heart disease, and cancer later in life. A 1994 study in *Epidemiology* reported this largely unheralded fact: Women who were breastfed as babies, even if only for a short time, have a lower risk of developing either premenopausal or postmenopausal breast cancer than do women who were formula-fed as babies. In general, scientists have found that the protection afforded by breast milk is greatest when formula feeding is excluded; this protection declines in proportion to the degree of supplementation with formula.

The Benefits of
Breastfeeding for Mothers

Does breastfeeding have any benefits for you, the mother, besides the pleasures of having a healthy, happy baby? Would nature have designed it otherwise? Breastfeeding affords an astonishing array of maternal benefits, both physical and emotional, and short- and long-term.

During and after birth, your body produces the hormone oxytocin to initiate the let-down of your milk. Your baby's suckling stimulates the production and release of oxytocin. The hormone simultaneously stimulates your uterus to contract; the contractions help to control blood loss and to return your uterus to its size before pregnancy. The hormone prolactin, also secreted when your nipples are stimulated, suppresses ovulation as long as you nurse your baby frequently. In countries where babies are customarily nursed for two to four years, breastfeeding functions as an essential birth-control method, guaranteeing that every baby receives sufficient nutrients and protection against disease before the next baby is born, and that the mother is not overtaxed by too-frequent childbearing.

Breastfeeding reduces a woman's risk of breast cancer. As the *New England Journal of Medicine* states, "If women who do not breastfeed or who breastfeed for less than three months were to do so for four to twelve months, breast cancer among parous premenopausal women (women of childbearing age who have given birth at least once) could be reduced by 11 percent; if all women with children lactated for 24 months or longer, the incidence might be reduced by nearly 25 percent." Although research has turned up a host of factors that influence a woman's risk of breast cancer, breastfeeding is clearly one of the most significant. In populations where breastfeeding is the norm, the incidence of breast cancer is minimal. Among the Tanka of South China, who traditionally nurse their babies with their right breasts only, 80 percent of the breast cancer that develops in older women occurs in their left breasts, on which their babies never nursed. The exact mechanism by which breastfeeding thwarts cancer is unknown. It seems clear, however, that when our breasts are allowed to function as they are meant to, they are healthier and stay healthier.

Breastfeeding has been found to provide increased protection for women against other cancers, too, including uterine, cervical, and ovarian. Women who have breastfed are less likely to develop rheumatoid arthritis than women who have not. Diabetic women who breastfeed have decreased insulin requirements while they're nursing, and women who breastfeed are less likely to develop diabetes at any point in their adult life. They are also 25 percent less likely to get osteoporosis as are women who formula-feed, and they tend to have fewer urinary tract infections.

Breastfeeding burns calories—more than 600 per day for women who don't give their babies formula supplements. In one study, mothers who breastfed exclusively or partially had, on average, lost more fat around their hips and were closer to their prepregnancy weights at three months postpartum than mothers who fed only formula.

And, as nursing mothers will tell you in chorus, breastfeeding has the most marvelous calming effect on them. A recent study documents their experience: At one month postpartum, breastfeeding women were significantly less anxious than formula-feeding women. The breastfeeding hormones, oxytocin and prolactin, cause a feeling of well-being that tends to promote maternal behavior. Also, the act of breastfeeding requires a woman to relax. No matter how hectic her life, a breastfeeding mother must sit or lie down with her baby eight or more times a day. And we mustn't discount the simple joy and peace of mind that come with cuddling a secure, satisfied, comfortable baby.

Whether or not they care that nursing is good for their health, most experienced nursing mothers would say that breastfeeding's primary benefit is convenience. Although breastfed babies nurse more frequently than do formula-fed babies, the non-nursing mother must dedicate a great deal of time to purchasing and mixing formula, cleaning bottles and nipples, and warming bottles. Unlike formula, breast milk is always ready, warm, and, as long as the baby continues to nurse frequently, plentiful. When the baby is hungry, the breastfeeding mother simply finds a comfortable place to settle down with him. At night, whereas the formula-feeding parent must wake up and get out of bed to prepare a bottle, the breastfeeding mother can have her baby brought to her, or, if her baby is sharing her bed, nurse without ever fully waking up. A breastfed baby is also highly portable: There are no bottles to pack and carry; there is no need to find a place to mix formula and heat the bottle. A spare diaper in her purse, and the breastfeeding mother and her baby are on their way.

The Benefits of Breastfeeding for Working Mothers

Many women going back to work decide that the "added stress" of nursing is the last thing they need. Whatever their reasons for not wanting to combine nursing and working, women who intend to return to work are more likely to wean early and less likely to initiate breastfeeding at all.

If they do nurse, however, and continue past their return to work, they may discover that their lives are made easier rather than harder by breastfeeding. One experienced mother finds that "breastfeeding is the easier part of being a working mother. It's much harder finding time to iron a shirt."

The immunologic properties of breast milk benefit working parents as much as their babies. Breastfed babies wake their parents less often at night with earaches and stuffy noses. Because breastfed babies are generally healthier, they also tend to be happier. They cry less, smile more, and are less wearying to care for after a long day at work.

The anti-infective properties of breast milk are a real boon when a baby is or will be in group daycare. Babies in daycare are exposed to more germs than are babies cared for at home. But when these babies are breastfed, they are protected against many serious bacterial and viral infections and secondary complications. The lower incidence and severity of illness in breastfed babies reduces the time their parents must take off from work.

The flood of relaxation that comes with the let-down of milk is made to order for working mothers. You may find that, after nursing your baby at the end of the day, you have trouble remembering what had so vexed you at work just a few hours earlier. Your slate is wiped clean, and you can more easily and calmly attend to your family and yourself for the rest of the evening. A pediatrician comments, "My greatest release after coming home is putting up my feet and nursing the baby. We both feel wonderful. It is my unwinding time."

For the typical nursing and working mother, the most important benefit of breastfeeding is that day after day it confirms that she is irreplaceable to her baby. Most women who decide to breastfeed do so for their babies' sakes. Only later do they discover that it's good for them, too. For working mothers, breastfeeding is a friend, a constant ally against the anxiety that comes from having to leave their babies in someone else's care for most of the day, and wondering if they are good-enough mothers. For your baby, after all, the babysitter may be very nice, but only Mama has a soft, sweet-smelling breast and warm, sweet-tasting milk. And when you pick up the baby and nurse at the end of a workday, you and she are immediately a couple again. There is no "getting to know you again" period for a working mother and her nursing baby.

A physician says, "Nursing has been a wonderful way to reconnect with my children while working. My daughter's favorite time to nurse is right after I get home at the end of the day. Even though she now goes all day without nursing, she gets a little frantic once I get home, and she really wants to nurse. I have found that nursing puts life into perspective. The sense of accomplishment, bonding, and well-being that I get from nursing makes me less anxious about having to leave her during the day."

A book editor concurs. "I like that it keeps me feeling connected to him all day long. I'm forced to take 'baby time' when I'm at work, and I can even go see him in the middle of a workday if I want. It helps ease the transition for me to nurse him when I drop him off and when

I pick him up. I also feel like I'm still mothering him even when I'm not with him, by continuing to provide pumped breast milk for him."

A social worker who formula-fed her first baby and breastfed her second speaks poignantly of the difference: "Since my mother-in-law took care of my first child for eight to ten hours a day, and could feed him just as well as I could, sometimes I felt as though he was more hers than mine. Since I had to be away from him 40 hours a week, breastfeeding could have tied us back together at the end of the day. Not breastfeeding my son is one of the greatest regrets of my life. My experience with him made me determined to have a different experience when my daughter was born."

Breastfeeding after returning to work is a way to tie the two halves of your life together. It will help you to make sense of yourself in the challenging new role as mother while continuing your pre-baby work life. Learning the job of motherhood is hard enough without the distractions of responsibilities outside the home, but when you're trying to maintain your identity as a working woman you have an intensified need for the lessons taught by breastfeeding. You can rely on breastfeeding as a blueprint for the intuitiveness, nurturing, and empathy that comes with experienced mothering. Through breastfeeding, you can give your child the best possible beginning, and in return you will gain confidence in yourself as a mother.

Parenting by Instinct

Once we consider all the aspects of breastfeeding—behavioral, immunologic, and nutritive—we cannot help but be impressed by how perfectly we humans have evolved to feed our babies. This may lead us to wonder what other special baby-care behaviors have evolved with our species. If you traveled now to societies that are still much the same as they have been for thousands of years, what would you see? How do parents take care of babies in cultures unchanged by such technological marvels as the clock, the baby bottle, and the baby carriage?

Ethologists, or researchers in the biologic bases of human behavior, have studied traditional cultures in every part of the world. They have identified a collection of ways in which parents all over the world care for their babies. These ways can be assumed to be humankind's basic parenting practices—practices that have evolved with our species. Like breast milk, they are perfectly matched to the needs of the human baby.

In every traditional society we know about, mothers keep their babies with them most of the time, from the moment of birth on. In the first hours after birth, they hold their babies skin-to-skin against their breasts and abdomens. They breastfeed within those first hours, and continue nursing until their babies are ready to wean or another baby is born or expected. As babies in traditional societies tend to be spaced three or four years apart, each baby may nurse until he is three or four. Mothers in these societies tend to respond to their babies' cries quickly and without fear of "spoiling" them. They carry or "wear" their babies for most of each day, while they accomplish the work of their day, unless someone else in the family or village is carrying or playing with baby. They are likely to sleep with their babies at night. These are the ways in which human beings have nurtured their babies since the beginning of time.

Pediatrician William Sears and his wife, Martha, a nurse, studied parenting styles among hundreds of families in southern California. They paid particular attention to those parents who seemed to enjoy raising children and whose children seemed to be turning out well. From their observations, the Searses developed a list of parenting practices that work well. Their list happens to be composed of the very same five practices that researchers have observed among parents in so many traditional cultures: holding babies skin-to-skin immediately after birth, breastfeeding until babies wean themselves, quickly responding to babies' cues, "wearing" babies, and co-sleeping.

The renowned naturalist Jane Goodall, for the lack of a better role model in her jungle-based research station, decided to care for her baby as some of our closest cousins, the chimpanzees, do theirs.

What did she do? She carried her baby with her wherever she went. She let him sleep in her bed. She responded quickly to his cues, as she had seen mother chimps do, and she breastfed him. As Jean Liedloff, an author who lived for several years with the Yequana Indians of South America and admired their gentle, skillful parenting (consisting of the same five practices), observes, "We have had exquisitely precise instincts, expert in every detail of child care, since long before we became anything resembling *Homo sapiens.*"

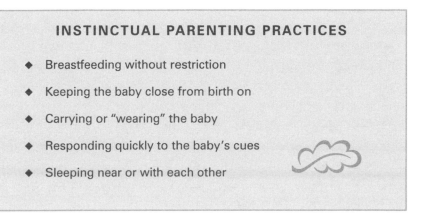

INSTINCTUAL PARENTING PRACTICES

◆ Breastfeeding without restriction

◆ Keeping the baby close from birth on

◆ Carrying or "wearing" the baby

◆ Responding quickly to the baby's cues

◆ Sleeping near or with each other

As modern "civilized" parents, we are deluged with new "proven" strategies for taking care of our babies, from bottle feeding on a schedule to letting them cry for hours so that they learn to fall asleep alone. We try out every new theory in hopes that it will ease this job of being a parent, the hardest we've ever known. Perhaps we are searching for answers because we have forgotten what we once knew so well. Perhaps being a parent is not supposed to be so hard.

Does this mean that, if you want to be the mother you were evolved to be, to care for your baby perfectly, you must sleep with her, carry her at all times, jump every time she peeps, and never be separated from her, beginning with the moment of birth? No, of course not. Mothers in traditional societies think of these practices not as rigid rules but just as what comes naturally most of the time. These mothers are simply doing what feels right. And, remember, they have many helping hands with both baby care and other kinds of work. A baby in these kin-based societies is passed around all day long from her mother to her father to her siblings to her cousin's husband's mother, showered with love as she goes. Few American mothers live in a harmonious, helpful extended family. But if you're hearing conflicting advice about the "right" way to care for your baby, it is useful to know what mothers knew before anyone thought to tell them anything at all.

This knowledge is especially useful when you are going back to work and wish to minimize the effect of each day's separation on your relationship with your baby. You can draw from this ancient pool of mothering knowledge to stay close to your baby. Think of these five practices—staying together, breastfeeding for a year or more, responding sensitively and quickly to your baby's cues, carrying or "wearing" your baby, and keeping your baby near or with you at night—as tools in your parenting toolbox. You may not use them all, or use them all the time, but you may find one or two especially handy. If you and your baby were not able to be together for the first hours or even days after birth, or if letting your baby sleep in your bed is unappealing, it's okay. Human evolution has provided you with an array of ways to ensure that you and your baby stay closely bonded. Nature has oversupplied mothers and babies to ensure that at least some of these practices take place, and that bonding is the result. The fact that you, like mothers through time, will also be working each day need make no difference at all. When and how these instinctual parenting practices may be of use to you in staying close to your baby will be discussed in the following chapters.

three

BREASTFEEDING BASICS

"*I never saw a baby nursing
until I nursed my own.***"**

LIKE MOTHERING IN GENERAL, breastfeeding is a learned art requiring practice and, usually, help from women who have successfully breastfed their own babies. Ideally, learning to breastfeed begins when you are breastfed yourself and continues as you grow up watching mothers in your family and community nurse their babies. Even chimpanzees that are raised in captivity without other chimps around them must be shown how to hold their babies and how to nurse them. In higher primates, including humans, the knowledge of how to feed our infants relies more on experience and observation than on instinct.

Most Western women who have grown up in the past 50 years have only occasionally, if ever, seen babies put to the breast. In the 1950s, 1960s, and early 1970s, few women breastfed at all, and although breastfeeding has regained popularity since then, many women still refuse to nurse in public or even in front of family members. So young women and girls have been unable to learn the art of breastfeeding as primates are designed to, by watching their elders. To confound matters, women's magazines, toy stores, and television are full of bottle-feeding images. A nursing mother was taken aback when her toddler, "who had never had a bottle in his mouth," suggested that a visitor's fussy baby might feel better if he were given a bottle. Researchers studying breastfeeding rates in Hispanic families have tracked a decline in breastfeeding and an increase in early weaning across generations. Rates of breastfeeding are high among Mexican mothers who have recently arrived to live in the United States. The longer the mothers live here, the less likely they are to breastfeed. Their American-born daughters have even lower rates, and their granddaughters are only as likely to nurse their babies as any other American. Culture is a pervasive and powerful influence; it sinks into our behavior more deeply than we might assume.

If you have not grown up watching nursing mothers, if you were not breastfed yourself, or if you tried to nurse a previous baby and could not, take time now to learn all you can about nursing from experienced mothers and, if possible, a professional lactation consultant. You may wish to attend a La Leche League (LLL) meeting in your community. An international organization of nursing mothers helping nursing mothers, LLL can be an invaluable source of accurate and empathetic breastfeeding advice. As a working mother, however, you may find some LLL leaders and meetings oriented to stay-at-home moms rather than mothers with jobs. If you don't feel comfortable in the first LLL meeting you attend, or if you find that the first leader you speak with on the phone seems unsupportive of working mothers, try another group or another leader, since each group has its own unique character. Unfortunately, LLL has acquired a reputation for hostility toward working mothers who rely on substitute caregivers. In fact, only a minority of LLL members are dogmatically opposed to maternal employment. LLL leaders are dedicated to helping all mothers, whether they are going back to work or not, and are glad to provide the one-on-one breastfeeding assistance that can make all the difference in the world. You can reach an LLL leader by telephone or through the Internet (see Resources, page 215).

Several excellent general books on breastfeeding are listed in the Resources section of this book. Although this book will give you all the basics on getting a good start in breastfeeding, other books can tell you how to handle special situations. Attend a breastfeeding class while you are pregnant, if possible. Educate your mate along with yourself; his support and enthusiasm for breastfeeding may be the key to your success.

The Very Beginning

For the best start in breastfeeding, nurse as soon after birth as your baby is ready. Researchers believe that the first hours after birth offer an optimal opportunity (although not the only one) for a mother and baby to establish a strong emotional attachment. Babies tend to be strikingly alert during the first hour after birth, a time when their parents are very eager to interact with them. Numerous studies have demonstrated the lasting benefit of this initial socializing. One study revealed that mothers who held their babies for the first hour after birth spoke more to their children even a full two years later than did mothers who were separated from their babies during the first hour. The mothers who had had the early contact asked twice as many questions of their toddlers as the control group of mothers did, and gave fewer commands. Asking questions is a sign of a harmonious relationship; commands express aggressive dominance. Another study showed that mothers who socialized with their babies right after birth felt more competent and less anxious than mothers who were separated from their babies. Yet another study revealed that babies who were held skin-to-skin by their mothers in the first hour calmed more easily and cried less in the first month than babies who were not.

Babies display a readiness to suck during the first two hours after birth that is not as strong again until forty hours later. If you nurse soon after birth, your baby's sucking will help contract your uterus by stimulating release of the hormone oxytocin. Besides planting the seed for a powerful and lasting emotional attachment, your first contact with your baby can help ensure your physical health.

Although most hospitals no longer routinely separate mothers and babies after birth, you may still need to state your preferences on the matter. Let your doctor and the hospital staff know that you intend to nurse as soon as possible after giving birth, whether in the delivery room after a vaginal birth or in the recovery room after a cesarean section.

If you plan to but in the end cannot spend the first hour of life holding your baby and initiating breastfeeding, don't fret. While it is a ripe opportunity to get off to a good start, mothers and babies are too drawn to each other not to make up for it at other times a little later. As soon as you and your baby are ready, lots of skin-to-skin holding and cuddling and nursing will feel right and do you both good. You have much time ahead of you to get to know and love your baby. Breastfeeding, carrying your baby, and keeping him near you at night will be especially helpful for the two of you.

While you're in the hospital, plan on "rooming in," or keeping your baby in your room with you rather than in the nursery. Ask the hospital staff in advance whether you will need a private room if you're to keep your baby with you both day and night. If the hospital does not seem to support rooming in, or a nurse says, "Yes, you can have your baby with you except during the night or when the doctors are on the floor," you may want to investigate any other hospitals or birthing centers that may be available to you. Or ask your baby's pediatrician to write an order on your chart for full-time rooming-in.

Contrary to what many people believe, new mothers who keep their babies with them 24 hours a day become no more fatigued than do mothers whose babies stay in the nursery. After all, you can doze and nurse at the same time, as you never could do while holding a bottle. Rooming-in allows you to feed your baby whenever and for however long both you and he wish, day and night, which is the very best way to guarantee a bountiful milk supply in the days to come. He will cry much less with you than he would in the nursery, too.

Keeping your baby with you means that you will know him better and feel more confident caring for him when the time comes to leave the hospital. You'll be less likely to experience the astonished panic so many parents recall on discharge. Establishing your trust in yourself as a competent mother right from the beginning will be the greatest gift you can give yourself, your baby, and your family in the days ahead.

> "Wait, are they going to let me just walk off with him? I don't know beans about babies!"
>
> —ANNE TYLER

Getting Started

Your nurse or midwife may help you put your baby to the breast for the first time. To begin, you will need to know a few basic facts about breastfeeding.

Proper positioning of your baby at the breast is the most important way to prevent or reduce nipple soreness, stimulate your milk production, and ensure a good milk supply for weeks or months to come. The "crossover hold" is the easiest way to get started: Hold the baby with the arm opposite from the breast you're starting with, support her neck and head with your hand, and position her face directly in front of your breast. Use pillows wherever you need them to prop up your baby, your arm, or both. Your baby should not have to turn her head to reach your nipple with her mouth—and you should not have to lean over to reach her mouth with your nipple. For complete images of proper positioning at the breast, go online to La Leche

League's Web site: www.lalecheleague.org. Search "positioning and latch on."

Next, let your baby latch on to your nipple only when her mouth opens very wide, as if she were yawning. Squeeze a few drops of colostrum onto her lips, or tickle her lips with your nipple, to get her interested. As soon as she opens wide, pull her close so that the tip of

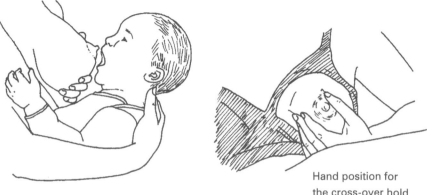

Cross-over hold

Hand position for
the cross-over hold

her nose just touches your breast. Don't lean over her, but bring her to you. Press her firmly to your breast; babies' noses, turned up and slightly flared, are able to breathe even when pressed against a breast. Cup your breast with your free hand to support it.

If your baby is sucking just the nipple rather than as much of your areola as her mouth can hold, she is not latched on properly. Take her off and try again. Remember, you are both learning this dance together. As your baby nurses, your nipple should be drawn to the rear of her throat and her gums should be around your areola. You know your baby is properly latched on when she has taken in an inch or more of the lower areola in her mouth (more of the bottom of the areola should be in her mouth than the top) and when her chin and the tip of her nose are touching your breast. Check to see that your baby's lips are relaxed outward, like fish lips, rather than tucked in. You will also know that your baby is latched on well if you are comfortable.

Before taking your baby off the breast, watch for cues that she has finished. Generally, a baby will let go of the breast on her own, and often she'll fall asleep. When you switch her to the other side, hold her upright to give her a chance to burp out any air she may have swallowed (not all babies burp after each feeding). As she awakens a little, switch her to the other side to suck some more.

If you do wish to take your baby off the breast before she lets go on her own, break the suction between her mouth and your nipple by slipping your finger into the corner of her mouth. Pulling a baby off without breaking the suction first can stretch the nipple and make it sore.

Even if you can't feel your milk letting down, you can tell when it does by watching your baby's sucking rate. Her quick, short sucks will change to a steady pattern of one or two long, drawing sucks followed by a swallow, and a little wiggle at her ears and temples.

Two to five bowel movements a day, after the third day, and mustard-colored stools by the fifth day of life, will confirm that your baby is latching on and sucking well. A lack of daily stools or stools that by the fifth day are still very dark suggest that a baby may not be latching on well and drawing sufficiently. Talk to a lactation consultant at your hospital or pediatrician's office if you are not seeing a change in the color of your baby's stools.

Hospital nurses and pediatricians sometimes recommend that you limit the first nursings to 5 minutes on each breast, then gradually increase the time to 10 and then 15 minutes. This is supposed to prevent sore nipples, but it doesn't. Nursing on-again-off-again is, in fact, likely to cause sore nipples. Besides, most newborns need to suck for 5 minutes just to get started. If your baby is positioned correctly and latched on well, there is no need to watch the clock.

After the first few feedings, try nursing in other positions—lying down or holding your baby's tummy against your tummy. With frequent nursings (every two hours or more), you will find after a few weeks that you hardly have to think about positioning and latch-on at all; both you and your baby will settle into a correct position naturally and comfortably whether you are sitting up or lying down—or, as time goes by, talking on the phone or working at the computer.

When you've finished your first nursing, you've accomplished your first lesson in sensitive mothering. From this moment forward, your baby's cues, and your growing child's cues, are your best guide to your own actions as his mother. Watch your baby, not the clock. Listen to your own feelings, not your neighbor's or your mother-in-law's opinions. Breastfeeding will teach you to read your baby's subtle, unspoken language. The sensitivity you thus acquire will be the foundation of a deep attachment and harmonious relationship between mother and child—a relationship that cannot be disrupted even by daily separations when you return to work.

Minimizing Engorgement

Your milk will come in gradually, beginning, probably, on the second or third day after birth. When you feel your breasts getting fuller you should nurse frequently, even if you have to wake the baby to do so. This will minimize engorgement, which occurs when the breasts fill with milk until they become larger and firmer, in some cases astonishingly big and hard. Your breasts are not intended to store milk, but they will hold some, if it is not withdrawn, while you become increasingly uncomfortable. Engorgement can also make latching-on a challenge for your baby. Frequent nursings right from the beginning will turn your colostrum to mature milk quickly, help you to manage the temporary engorgement that most mothers experience in the first week, and make it easier for your baby to latch on to your nipples.

Avoiding Sore Nipples

Breastfeeding is not supposed to hurt. Nevertheless, sore nipples are so common that they are sometimes considered inevitable. Tender nipples in the first few days after birth are normal. As your baby latches on and stretches the nipple into her mouth, you'll feel a pinch that passes as your milk lets down. A dose of ibuprofen or acetaminophen a half hour before nursing will minimize this early tenderness. Usually by the end of the second week, if the baby is positioned and sucking well, the pinch will be gone altogether.

Truly sore nipples, however, may be damaged or abraded and need help healing. They are a sign that a baby may not be latching on properly. If your nipples are sore beyond that initial pinch, allow them to air-dry between nursings, and avoid wearing a bra (especially while sleeping). Lanolin and glycerin or hydrogel dressings for sore nipples, available at some pharmacies and through lactation consultants, can be very soothing. Don't limit your baby's nursing time; frequently putting the baby on and taking him off the breast may aggravate the problem, besides upsetting the baby.

For advice on healing sore and cracked nipples, see page 66.

Seeking Help

If your nipples become exceedingly sore or if your baby has difficulty latching on and staying on the breast, seek the help of a professional lactation consultant. Do this *before* you leave the hospital, if possible. Many maternity floors now have a lactation consultant on staff; the nurses will ask her to stop by your room if you request it. Sometimes there is an unhelpful delay between your request and the arrival of the lactation consultant, because she is on a part-time schedule or has too heavy a patient load. It's wise to make your request to see her as early as possible, even if you're not having a problem, to confirm that all is well. Later, you may be able to visit a breastfeeding clinic, or even hire a lactation consultant to visit you at home. Or you can consult with a local La Leche League leader. Early observation and guidance by an expert can keep most breastfeeding problems from becoming serious. Beware of accepting casual advice from friends, relatives, or even pediatricians and nurses who haven't studied lactation or breastfed successfully themselves. "You may not be making enough milk," they may tell you. "Why don't you give the baby a bottle, just this time?" Careful observation will reveal the cause of whatever problem you are having (not having enough milk is one of the *least* likely), and an experienced, informed person can help you find its solution.

How Your Breasts Produce Milk

If you are planning to go back to your job within a few weeks or months, you may be wondering how being away from your baby for hours each day will affect breastfeeding. Understanding how and when your breasts produce milk will enable you to manage your milk supply and meet your baby's nutritional needs.

When your nipples are stimulated, your brain releases the hormones prolactin and oxytocin, which in turn cause your breasts to secrete and release milk. Prolactin is the milk-producing hormone. The more frequently and effectively your baby sucks, the more prolactin your body releases and the more milk your breasts produce. Oxytocin is the milk-ejection hormone. It contracts the sacs where milk is made to push the milk through ducts to the nipple. This sudden release of milk is your "let-down reflex." Your baby takes milk from your breast by sucking, but you are also giving milk by letting it down. Both actions are required for successful breastfeeding. In the early weeks of breastfeeding a vigorous let-down can eject milk with hilarious gusto, spraying it in twin fountains. When let-down occurs, the baby hardly needs to milk the breast; the milk is pumped into her throat. Your milk may let down several times in the course of a feeding.

Letting down your milk is crucial to your baby's nutrition. The milk that is stored in the breasts and can be drawn out by sucking alone is low in fat. It may satisfy your baby's need for fluid and is perfect for times when your baby is only thirsty or just nursing for comfort. After the milk lets down, however, comes your baby's wonderfully satiating square meal—milk that is held in the cells farther back in your breast and gets creamier as the feeding progresses. Dr. F. E. Hytten, of the University of Aberdeen in Scotland, has demonstrated with the help of sponges that fat particles in breast milk tend to cling to the walls of the alveoli and ducts and to be drawn off last. The baby's last few swallows of milk from the first breast sucked contain the most fat of all (assuming your milk lets down during the nursing, and the baby releases the breast herself when she is satiated). The fat mixes more evenly in the second breast, although some gradation remains. Dr. Michael Woolridge identified several English babies who were failing to gain weight because their mothers had been firmly told to nurse only 10 minutes on each breast at each feeding; following that rule, the mothers were feeding their babies on what was effectively skim milk.

A good breast pump stimulates let-down just as your baby does. Being able to let down your milk in response to the stimulation of your pump, as well as to your baby, is essential if you are to collect significant amounts of milk after you return to work.

In the early months, your milk may let down anytime you are reminded of your baby. You might be talking to a friend on the phone, telling her about the baby, and suddenly feel the tingle of your milk letting down and spreading dampness in your bra and blouse. The sound of your baby's cry may bring down your milk in a gush. When you begin pumping your milk at work, you may find that you can prompt your let-down reflex by looking at a picture of your baby as you pump or by breathing in the scent of a nightie your baby wore the night before. You may even associate the pump itself with your baby, and so find your milk letting down as soon as you get out the pump.

The let-down reflex can also be conditioned to occur at certain times during the day. If your baby settles into a regular feeding pattern, his meal may be ready and dripping before you even put him to the breast. In the same way, when you begin pumping your milk at work, you may find your milk letting down as soon as you turn the lock in the door of the room in which you pump.

In time the system settles down; leaking and spraying will soon become a memory of newborn days. Until then, add a collection of cotton breast pads to your nursery supplies, and tuck a couple into your nursing bra each day.

Establishing Your Milk Supply

Breastfeeding is a supply-and-demand system; that is, your breasts produce milk in response to sucking. When there is more sucking (by a well-positioned baby or a good pump), they produce more milk; when there is less sucking, they make less milk. If ever you feel that your milk production is tapering off, simply increase the number of times you put your baby to the breast each day and, if necessary, pump your milk just after nursing or an hour or two after your baby begins a long sleep stretch. Frequent short nursings (20-minute sessions every two hours or so) will be more effective than longer but less frequent sessions.

> The law of supply and demand: The more you nurse your baby (or pump your milk), the more milk your body will produce.

As a working mother, you may notice fluctuations in your milk supply more than other mothers do. You may see your milk supply decrease over the course of the work week, build back up over the weekend, be quite plentiful on Monday, and then gradually decrease again as the week proceeds. Because you understand breastfeeding as a supply-and-demand system, you will know what to expect—and how to manage it. Specific techniques for managing your milk supply are described in Chapter 6.

Going Home

These days you are likely to be sent home from the hospital a day or two after your baby is born or, if you've had a cesarean section, on the third day. Your milk probably won't have come in yet. If your baby has been sleepy she may not have nursed very much yet. Sixty years ago, mothers and babies stayed in the hospital one to two weeks after delivery. Being sent home then meant that the mother and baby were deemed to have learned all the basics (of bottle-feeding, at least) and were ready to be on their own. But, these days, when a mother with 48 hours of experience is discharged with a 48-hour-old baby, it is not because they are necessarily well prepared to go home, but because insurance companies have found a dandy way to save money.

Of course many mothers are happy to leave the hospital as soon as possible, thereby avoiding the rules, schedules, separations from their babies, and supplementary feedings of glucose water or formula that once were standard in every hospital and still are in many. (Even in a large hospital known for its outstanding maternity care, in 2005 a new mother was urged by a nurse to give her healthy breastfed baby a bottle of formula because the baby was "such a big girl.") But going home without the support you need there can be as challenging as avoiding hospital interventions.

In recent years, somehow, American mothers have grown fond of the myth of the pioneer woman who planted fields in the morning, gave birth without assistance to a healthy baby at midday, and spent the rest of the afternoon baking bread. If those women could do it, the moral is, so can we, in our modern way: We can work up until the day before labor, go to the hospital and give birth, then come home and call work. A 1985 guide to pregnancy and birth for career women exalts the advertising executive who "felt so ready to go back to work that she met her housekeeper in the lobby of the hospital and let her take the baby home while [she] went back to the office." Even new mothers who resist the pressure to "do it all" may believe in the myth of the woman who gave birth while plowing the field, and feel that they are not living up to our culture's expectations.

In past centuries and in other societies there are and have always been stringent rules and rituals for taking care of new mothers and babies; some societies still have such rules and rituals. These traditions have worked to keep the mother well and rested and nourished and to strengthen the attachment that can ensure an infant's survival. In Jamaica and many other places, the midwife stayed on for a few days after birth to look after any other children and to do the cooking or washing for the family, so that the mother could rest and focus on her new baby. In rural southern India, a mother stayed with her newborn in a special hut for 90 days, visited only by her husband and midwife. Among the Hopi, a mother and baby remained in a darkened room for 18 days. The Lummi of the Northwest coast required a 12-day seclusion period for mother, baby, and father, all of whom were attended by the "helping women." In ancient Japan, both parents and their newborns were secluded for 35 days, and even today Japanese babies are rarely taken out of the home before they are a month old. In most societies, a new mother is still fed special foods to make her strong and her milk bountiful. "Thus the initial learning time in which mother and baby become attached to each other is safeguarded and given special ritual significance by the culture," writes Sheila Kitzinger, social anthropologist and author of numerous books on birth and motherhood. Women in traditional societies go back to work, of course, but only after their transition to motherhood is well begun.

There is no doubt a biological basis to these worldwide postpartum traditions. Prolactin, the milk-making hormone, is highest in a mother's bloodstream for the first 40 days after delivery. Prolactin levels then decline, though very gradually, as the mother continues breastfeeding. How then do many women continue nursing their babies for two years or more, past the point when prolactin disappears from their systems? What keeps up the milk-making process? One hypothesis is that the high levels of prolactin generated by exclusive breastfeeding in the first six weeks may somehow enable the breasts to work independently of the prolactin stimulus after this period. Perhaps ancient peoples understood that a generous confinement period helped a mother establish her milk supply. They may have noticed a better survival rate in infants who were secluded with their mothers.

Kittie Frantz, a widely respected pediatric nurse practitioner, put this hypothesis into practice in Santa Monica, California. Approximately 90 percent of her patients were working, nursing mothers, and nearly all of them complained that they had difficulty maintaining their milk supplies when they went back to work. The common practice in the area was to begin pumping and feeding pumped milk to babies at two weeks of age to get them used to a bottle early on. Frantz began to recommend freezing the pumped milk and delaying bottle feeding until a baby was four to five weeks old. The babies received no supplements or breast milk by bottles until the first month was past. When her patients followed this advice, their success in maintaining bountiful milk supplies was, Frantz says, "phenomenal." These mothers would ask her, "Why do I have so much milk for my baby when all my friends are struggling?" Her answer: "We heeded the wisdom of the women who came before us."

Safeguard the first six weeks or so after giving birth to your baby. It is your babymoon. Before the baby is born, preferably, ask your mother or your mother-in-law, a sister or a dear friend, to come and help out—not only with the baby but with meals, housekeeping, and caring for your other children, if this is not your first baby. Ideally, this helper—or "doula," as such a person is often called—will also be experienced in breastfeeding, or at least supportive of it. The father, of course, may take this role, but it is the rare husband who can take more than a week off work to help out at home or who brings more experience than the mother to baby care. Besides, a father should also have the opportunity to focus on his new child without the constant distraction of housework and cooking. Many grandmothers visit for a couple of weeks whenever a grandchild is born, to help the new mother so she can care for her new baby without distraction. One mother remembers her own mother's visit with a smile: "I never changed a diaper the first month. I never shopped or cooked or cleaned. I lived from feeding to feeding, every two hours."

Your mother or other relative may or may not support your decision to breastfeed. She may agree that breast is best, but contribute poor advice and misinformation to the process. A lack of good breast-feeding support is a primary reason that many women give up nurs-ing in the early days or weeks. Remember that, in the time and place your mother or mother-in-law gave birth, bottle feeding may have been standard practice and breastfeeding widely misunderstood. If she didn't nurse her babies, she may feel uncomfortable or even guilty now. She may have been looking forward to sharing the feed-ing of a grandchild, and may now feel disappointed.

If this is the case in your family, finding breastfeeding support and assistance from an experienced friend, a La Leche League leader, or a lactation consultant will be all the more essential. Call La Leche League or the International Lactation Consultant Association (see Resources, page 216) for a referral, or ask the nurses in your mater-nity ward for recommendations. Investigate postpartum support services in your area. Doulas-for-hire are now available in most major cities and their suburbs, and some provide lactation counseling as well as domestic help. Look in your local parents' paper, if there is one, for advertisements. You might consider hiring a postpartum service for the first three or four days after birth and asking a rela-tive to come and help when you first return to work (see Chapter 6 for more on this subject).

Accept all offers of help from friends and neighbors. If you don't know what help you'll need, say you'll call them, or have your mate or doula call them, once you are home with the baby. (What you don't need is a professional baby nurse to take care of the baby for you. If someone takes care of you, you can take care of your baby.) Anne Lamott, the writer and a single mother, remembers one night not long after her baby was born, when a visitor from her church, a man in his sixties, arrived at the door. "After exchanging pleasantries he said, 'I wanted to do something for you and the baby. So what I want to ask is, What if a fairy appeared on your doorstep and said that he or she would do any favor for you at all, anything you wanted around the house that you felt too exhausted to do by yourself and too ashamed to ask anyone else to help you with?'

"'I can't even say,' I said. 'It's too horrible.' But he finally convinced me to tell him, and I said it would be to clean the bathroom. He ended up spending an hour scrubbing the bathtub and toilet and sink with Ajax and lots of hot water. I sat on the couch while he worked, watching TV, feeling vaguely guilty and nursing Sam to sleep." Such kindly fairies are all too rare. We are not meant to enter into parenthood alone and without help.

On discharge from the hospital, you probably will be given a goodbye gift of baby-care pamphlets, perhaps tucked into a basket with a pair of booties or a rattle, a few disposable diapers, and a can of baby formula. Take the booties and the diapers, but leave the can of formula. Giving "formula kits" to all new mothers, including breastfeeding mothers, is a widespread hospital practice funded by formula manufacturers. The message is implicit that you need formula "just in case"–that breastfeeding is an experiment that may not work out. The formula manufacturers hope you will try out their product at some point in the early weeks–which is easy to do if it is sitting on your kitchen shelf–and thus begin the cycle of supplementation that so often leads to early weaning. But you won't face this temptation if you leave the bait behind.

Some mothers are surprised to find the trip home from the hospital exhausting. Be sure to go straight to bed, and tuck your baby in beside you. You need to rest so you'll retrieve your strength, and to nurse frequently to help your milk come in, if it hasn't already. Provided you have plenty of tender care by people who love you, home is the best place to establish lactation.

four

LIFE ON LEAVE:
THE FOURTH TRIMESTER

"*Breastfeeding lets me tell my baby
things with my body that she wouldn't
understand with words for a long time.***"**

Becoming a Mother

WHEN YOU GIVE BIRTH TO A BABY, you also give birth to a
mother. Expect the weeks and (with luck) the months of
your maternity leave to be an intense interval in your
life. Not only are you learning to understand and to answer your
baby's unique needs, but your sense of self is undergoing a tec-
tonic shift.

If this is your first baby, your inner task at this time is to integrate your identity as a mother into your established identity.
Women experience this process with varying degrees of ease
and upheaval. If you have built your self-image largely on your
work, and if you relish your independence, you may find this
new identity especially hard to embrace. To compound the difficulty, your work may demand that you prevent your personal

life from entering your professional life in any way. But, as Joyce Block, a psychologist, writes, "Motherhood is not an experience that is easily compartmentalized." As a mother, you are no longer a lone individual. Although the umbilical cord has been cut, you and your baby remain connected emotionally and, if you are breastfeeding, physically, for many months after birth. For your newborn, you are the world. He relies on you to anticipate his needs, to interpret his cries, and to protect and nurture him just as your womb has done for the preceding nine months. And you now see life through a new lens, a lens with your child's image indelibly etched on its surface.

Your emotional bond with your baby, already well begun, deepens by incalculable fathoms during these early months. This may be the most wonderful journey you've ever taken, and yet at times you may feel in over your head. Enter into this stage knowing that you will eventually emerge as yourself but with new, rich dimensions. Sometimes, during this period, your old life may seem distant and unrelated to your new state of existence. The tidal wave of changes may tower so high that you wish you could build a wall against it before you are overwhelmed and your life is forever altered beyond recognition. You may find yourself trying to prevent changes from occurring, or denying that they have occurred. Yes, you've had a baby, but other than that, you insist, everything is the same. The truth is that nothing is the same, nor will anything ever be quite the same again. Your task is now to build a new reality that incorporates your motherhood.

In many ways our culture encourages parents to ignore their instincts, which are thought to create bad, self-indulgent habits. Just about everything a mother does because she wants to, because it seems like the easiest thing to do, and because it makes her baby happy—whether picking up a baby when he cries, or breastfeeding without a schedule, or bringing a baby into the parents' bed to sleep—has been labeled a bad habit by one expert or another. Bringing the baby into bed to sleep beside you, because this is easier and more restful than putting the baby to sleep elsewhere, has come under particular scrutiny by the experts in recent years. The recommendations to new parents, even those by the best-intentioned, most authoritative American Academy of Pediatrics, are derived, in part, from number crunching the data of multiple studies rather than common sense and empathy for new families. Published scientific studies are generally based on solid data, but the interpretation of that data is too often influenced by cultural biases. As writer John Seabrook notes in his 1999 article on infant co-sleeping in the *New Yorker,* "Perhaps the American veneration for a night of unbroken sleep is another culturally determined prejudice, posing as science." Although experts' recommendations, and the scientific studies on which they are based, are a valuable resource as we strive to raise healthy, safe children, your sense of what is right for you and your baby will become finely tuned over the first weeks and months of motherhood. Trust that sense and rely on it. Researchers will probably produce another conclusion another day, and the media will again reduce the studies to headline directives for new parents and the rest of us.

If your judgment needs the backing of biologic evidence, your body provides it. When your baby cries and you feel the urge to go to him, to put him to your breast, the blood flow to your breast increases. Your body knows what to do and is already responding, even if your mind has been convinced to hesitate. Research confirms that your physical responsiveness to your baby's cues—whether crying, rooting, fussing, eye contact, or any other form of infant communication—is the most important contributor to your baby's physical, emotional, and intellectual development. Your quick responses tell your baby that his actions are meaningful, that he is a person whose needs matter. Your sensitive interactions guide and encourage his developing sense of self. Responding to your baby, picking him up and cuddling him when he cries, and putting him to your breast and soothing him, teaches him trust. He trusts you to meet his needs. This deep trust forms the core of his sociability and self-esteem as he grows.

If you attend to your baby's needs sensitively now, she is more likely to grow into someone who nurtures others readily and who is easy to be with. As Michael Schulman and Eva Mekler, psychologists and authors of *Bringing Up a Moral Child,* conclude of the results of one wide-scale study, "children who were treated with sensitivity and cooperation tend to be sensitive and cooperative in turn." Recent work by attachment researcher Mary Main suggests that the quality of a maternal-infant attachment may even be "transgenerational"; that is, the nature of a mother's attachment to her mother influences the quality of the attachment she develops with her own child. Obtained through a research tool called the Adult Attachment Interview, Main's data reveal that the way adults remember and work through their relationships with their own parents is a powerful predictor of their own parenting practices. In the days ahead, as you endeavor to keep work and family life in balance, you will want to spend your hours at home in positive interactions with your child rather than in struggles of will. Now is the time to establish a deep, immutable harmony.

Following your maternal instincts is as important to your development as it is to your baby's. Each interaction with your baby refines your mothering skills and enhances your understanding of your baby. Through caring for your baby, you will grow, too. Experienced mothers who enjoy mothering, whether employed or not, would urge you to open the floodgates. Wallow in your passion for your baby, and in hers for you. Holding yourself back from your baby, perhaps by subscribing to the notion that you must teach her independence now so that your eventual separations will be easier, will hamper the natural process of learning to be her mother. Throw yourself headlong into baby love instead, and you'll soon develop the intuitive knowledge and sensitivity that are essential to a harmonious mother-baby relationship. If we could offer you but one sentence to guide you as you combine motherhood and employment, it would be this: *What matters most is not the number of hours that you and your baby will be together or apart, it is the quality of your attachment with your baby and your confidence in yourself as a mother.*

Breastfeeding in the Early Weeks: The Learning Period

You and your baby will learn to breastfeed over the next six to eight weeks. The ease with which you do so will depend on your baby's temperament and your own understanding of breastfeeding and infant development. Individual babies vary as much as individual adults do; nevertheless, a few milestones are predictable. One is that by eight weeks postpartum breastfeeding will be second nature to both of you.

In the beginning, expect your baby to want to nurse about every two or three hours during the day and a few times during the night. Generally, new babies nurse 8 to 12 times, or more, every 24 hours, with no more than 4 hours passing between feedings. Such frequent feedings are necessary because breast milk is digested rapidly and the stomach of a newborn is very small, about the size of a walnut. Nursing as often as your baby wants will keep him content and you comfortable, and will build your milk supply to suit your baby's needs.

You will know your baby is hungry and ready to nurse—before he begins wailing—when he roots, turning his head and reaching toward your breast with his chin and mouth and sticking his tongue out or making sucking motions. Offering the breast whenever you see these signs is sometimes called "feeding on demand," meaning the baby is fed whenever he wants. A better term would be "feeding on request," meaning you don't wait until the desire becomes a demand before satisfying it.

You too can request to nurse if your breasts are feeling especially full. If your baby tends to be very quiet and sleepy during these early weeks, you may need to wake him to nurse more frequently than he would on his own. This can keep you from getting engorged and help maintain your milk supply. Your baby needs these frequent feedings even if he doesn't request them.

As your baby grows he will eventually stretch out the time between nursings and sleep in longer stretches at night. All babies do these things, but on their own individual timetables. If you delay nursings or nurse according to a fixed schedule, you may find that your baby is no longer growing as expected, and that he's very unhappy, too.

Milestones during the early weeks include periodic growth spurts. At approximately ten days after birth, at four to six weeks of age, around three months, and again at six months, babies experience sudden and rapid growth. After settling into some semblance of a routine, your baby may one day begin nursing much more frequently. He may seem insatiable. Many a mother has believed (or has been told) that her baby is hungry because she cannot make enough milk for him. But the baby's insatiability will last for just a day or two, until he has stimulated the production of the additional milk he needs to fuel his growth spurt. (Older children do this as well, as parents know who have observed a usually picky eight-year-old suddenly eat everything on his plate and then ask for more.) Your baby manages this simple yet brilliant system with the efficiency of a factory foreman. He sucks in one way to stimulate let-down, in another way to swallow the flood of milk that comes with let-down. He even prepares for his growth spurts by nursing as much as possible to obtain the added energy he will need.

The sudden change in your baby's appetite during these growth spurts may alarm you. Your baby wants to nurse all the time; he is famished, and fussy, all day long. You may worry that your milk supply has dropped off, and wonder if you should give the baby a bottle of formula. You may fear that his behavior is going to go on forever.

It's not. Your milk supply hasn't fallen off; it's just that your baby's needs have suddenly risen. He is nursing more often to build up your milk supply. All you need do is allow your baby and your breasts to readjust to one another by nursing your baby without restriction or supplementation. Of course, you may not get much *else* done for a couple of days as your baby nurses 12 to 18 times in 24 hours, but this is just another part of becoming a mother. (See Chapter 7 for advice on dealing with growth spurts once you are back at work.)

Sometimes a new baby will want to nurse again and again, every 20 to 40 minutes, for two or more hours. Called "cluster feeding," this type of nursing usually occurs at night during the first week or two after birth. After a cluster of feedings, a baby usually falls into a deep sleep. These marathon nursing sessions are nature's way of establishing breastfeeding early on.

The average duration of nursings varies among babies. Babies nurse in different ways, some in infrequent long bursts, some more often and for shorter periods. Your breasts will adapt to the rhythm of your particular baby, with the milk letting down strongly at first, and then repeatedly or intermittently, according to the baby's sucking patterns. In the early weeks, when your baby is still learning to suck efficiently, he may take quite a long time to withdraw the milk he needs. To avoid sore nipples and engorgement and ensure an ample milk supply, let your baby determine the length of each nursing.

How do you know when your baby is full? She will signal her satiety by relaxing her clenched fists, by giving that sweet little flash of a newborn smile, by releasing the nipple, and often by falling asleep. Or, if your let-down reflex is strong, her tiny tummy may be full (for an hour or so) after nursing on only one breast, and she may refuse the other. If your baby does this, just be sure to offer the full side first at the next feeding.

Even if your baby seems to be asleep, you should offer both breasts at each feeding, starting on the side where the previous feeding ended. Newborns may sleep through feedings they and your milk supply need. Your baby may wake up and nurse again when you switch her to the other side, especially if you burp her in between. Undress your baby by a layer or two to wake her gently, and cuddle her skin to skin. Lightly rubbing her back, stroking her scalp, playing pat-a-cake, and talking while making eye contact may also stimulate her enough to begin nursing.

Avoiding Supplements

Supplementary bottles of formula or sugar water can interfere with learning to breastfeed and establishing a milk supply. Healthy breast-fed babies don't need any fluids besides breast milk. Supplements can suppress your baby's appetite, making her less eager for the breast. Also, since artificial nipples require a different way of latching on and sucking, they sometimes confuse babies still learning to breastfeed. Fluids flow rapidly through bottle nipples with barely any effort on the part of the baby. If your baby gets accustomed to supplementary bottles in the early days, she may become frustrated and fuss when your milk does not flow the moment she feels your nipple in her mouth. Let your baby learn to withdraw milk from the breast before she experiences the freer flow of fluid through a bottle nipple. Once breastfeeding is established, you will be able to give your baby a bottle safely (see Introducing the Bottle, page 159).

How to Tell If Your Baby Is Getting Enough Milk

Mothers' most common concern during these first weeks is whether the baby is getting enough milk. Wouldn't it be nice if our breasts were translucent—if we could see the milk being made, watch as it flows down the ducts to collect in the milk sinuses behind the nipple, and lets down with a gush? Bottle feeding has the psychological advantage that the bottle's contents reassuringly disappear into the baby right before your eyes. Perhaps bottle feeding would never have become so popular if bottles were made of an opaque material. Never mind. You can be sure your baby is getting enough milk if—

◆ he nurses at least 8 times in 24 hours;

◆ you see and hear him swallowing, after every suck or two;

- by the fifth day after birth, the color of his stools changes to mustard yellow;

- he has clear, pale urine (rather than dark yellow);

- he has one or more bowel movements per day; and

- he gains at least an ounce per day from the fifth day of life.

Of course, there are always individual variations. After about six weeks, a breastfed baby who is getting plenty of milk may not have a bowel movement for a couple of days. Weight gain also is highly individual; some babies may grow in length rather than in weight at first. For the first three to four months of life, gaining less than an ounce a day indicates an inadequate milk intake. Thereafter, gaining a half ounce a day is considered adequate for most babies.

Leaking Milk

The first few weeks of breastfeeding can be a rather *wet* time, as your milk leaks and drips and sprays, sometimes when you least expect it. While your baby nurses on one breast, the other breast may leak or even spray milk. This is a wonderful sign—it shows that your let-down reflex is working, even if you don't feel the pins-and-needles sensation that usually occurs when milk lets down (some women never feel this sensation). Your milk may also let down when you are reminded of your baby or of nursing—when someone asks about your baby, when you hear your baby making sounds in her sleep, or even when you just sit down in the chair where you most often nurse your baby. The relaxing warmth of a shower may also stimulate let-down. Over the next few weeks, leaking should gradually lessen, though the problem may recur when you go back to work, especially when you are very full or miss a pumping session.

While you're leaking, breast pads of cloth or paper will keep your bra and clothing dry. Reusable, washable cotton pads are the first choice of women who prefer the feel of cloth next to their skin. These pads vary in how much liquid they absorb and how quickly they wick it away from the nipple. Disposable paper pads are also a good choice, although those that are layered with plastic to make them waterproof can keep your nipples moist. (Plastic-lined pads can also slow healing, if your nipples are sore. But if you can't risk leaking while you stand before a jury or wear surgical scrubs, you may definitely prefer plastic-lined pads for short periods.) Some disposable pads have an adhesive strip to anchor the pad to the inside of your bra. Others are slit halfway to the center of the pad, so the pad can mold to the shape of your breast. Very thin pads can be layered for extra absorption.

Breast pads are available in drugstores, supermarkets, and baby-supply stores, but to get cloth ones you may need to order online or from a baby-care catalog or make your own by cutting up diapers. Nursing pads of a new type called LilyPadz not only soak up leaking milk but also apply slight pressure on the nipple to stop the leaking. These washable silicone pads can be worn with or without a bra and can even be worn in a swimsuit. They can be reused for months.

During this leaky phase you may also need to take a small towel into bed with you at night.

Healing Sore Nipples

Nipple soreness, perhaps the most common problem faced by new nursing mothers, ranges from a bit of tenderness to searing pain that can discourage the most committed woman. Usually the cause of the problem is incorrect positioning or sucking. If you are not certain your baby is nursing correctly, call a lactation consultant or a La Leche League leader. She may need to watch you nurse your baby before she can diagnose the problem and help you correct it. Once the problem is identified and corrected, the soreness should disappear within a couple of days.

You can help to prevent sore nipples by keeping them dry and exposed to air as much as possible. If your nipples are already sore or cracked, however, moist healing is required to avoid scab formation.

Medical-grade lanolin (Pur Lan or Lansinoh), or glycerin or hydrogel pads, will soothe sore nipples and keep your nursing sessions as comfortable as possible. These products are available online, from lactation consultants, and at some pharmacies. Damaged nipples may develop staph and other infections, putting a mother at risk for mastitis. If your nipple is bleeding and sore, talk to your doctor about treating it with antibiotics as soon as possible.

Almost always worst when the baby first latches on, the soreness may lessen as the milk lets down. Always begin nursing on the side that is least sore; nursing on the other side will be less painful after the milk lets down. Nurse frequently, so that your baby does not come to the breast ravenous; a hungry baby can be hard on a sore nipple. Massaging your breasts or using a warm compress as you nurse may help your milk to let down more quickly. Taking a dose of an over-the-counter pain reliever, ibuprofen or acetaminophen, 20 minutes before nursing is safe for your baby and will also help to decrease the ouch of the initial latch on.

Nursing in a variety of positions can help minimize soreness by distributing the pressure rather than letting it fall on the same part of the nipple at each feeding. In all positions, make sure the baby comes straight onto the breast and that you are holding him close enough and high enough so that he doesn't drag the breast downward or have to tilt or twist his head to nurse.

Your nipples can also be made sore by a thrush infection. Thrush is caused by *Candida albicans*, a fungus that thrives on milk on the nipples, in the milk ducts, and in the baby's mouth. If your nipples suddenly become red and itchy or burning after the first week or more of breastfeeding, you may be dealing with a case of thrush. Other symptoms include cracked nipples and shooting pains in one or both breasts during or after a feeding. If you've got thrush, your baby most likely does, too. She may have white patches on the inside of her cheeks or lips or on the tongue, or a diaper rash. She may nurse reluctantly or with an altered suck because her mouth is sore.

If you suspect you have a thrush infection, see your doctor. She may prescribe liquid nystatin for your baby's mouth and nystatin cream for your nipples and areola. You can also treat your nipples with an over-the-counter anti-fungal such as Lotrimin. (Apply it after your baby nurses and wipe any residue off before the next nursing.) Continue treatment for two weeks, even though the symptoms will be gone in as little as a day or, at the most, five days. If you are using cloth breast pads, change and wash them after every feeding in hot, soapy water, and boil them every day for a few minutes. Rinse your nipples after nursing, and wash your hands frequently to avoid re-infection. You should of course keep nursing throughout the infection and its treatment; if nursing is too painful, pump the affected breast with a fully automatic breast pump.

Preventing and Treating Plugged Ducts and Breast Infections

If you notice a tender place in your breast, one that is especially sore when you press on it, it is very probably a plugged duct. Plugged ducts are less common than sore nipples, but can be even more dis-couraging. They are caused when a milk duct does not drain completely and the milk backs up and forms a plug. The plug puts pressure on the tissue around it, which becomes inflamed and sore. If the plug is not loosened, the tissue may become infected. Often a plugged duct is a message from your body to your brain saying, "You're doing too much. You need to rest *now.*"

Plugged ducts are truly tiresome. The best remedy, however, is not weaning but frequent nursing—at least every 2 hours for 24 hours or as long as the breast is tender. If you can, go straight to bed—*with* your baby. Start every feeding on the affected side, and vary the positions in which you nurse. Lactation consultants advise nursing the baby in a position that points his chin at the sore spot ("even if you have to stand on your head to do it," says one lactation consultant); that spot will then receive the most suction. Just pulling your baby's knees tight against your tummy will help, by evening the pressure against your breast. Warm, wet heat on the sore place can help dilate the duct. Massage the area gently while it is warm, pressing the lump toward your nipple. You are trying to knead the duct open so that the backed-up milk can flow freely again. Sometimes a plug is in a nipple pore; you may see dried secretions come out as a spaghetti-like strand or as dry, sandy bits. Either breastfeed your baby or pump your milk on the affected side immediately after massaging to further clear the plug. Taking a day off to rest, nurse frequently, and treat your breast with moist heat and gentle massage may well prevent a bout of mastitis.

> The Instaheat Pad is a nifty remedy for plugged ducts and mastitis. Made by Medela, the sealed plastic bag is filled with sodium acetate and water and contoured to fit into a bra over a sore spot. Bend the bag to set off a chemical reaction that causes the fluid inside to become hot. It can be reused by microwaving or boiling. The Instaheat Pad is available from online vendors.

If you have a very painful spot in your breast (one that is red, warm, and hard), if you have a fever, and if you ache all over as though you are coming down with the flu, you can be almost certain that you have developed a breast infection, or mastitis. If the fever is high or has lasted for more than 12 hours, you may need antibiotics. Call your doctor. Be cautious, however, if the doctor advises you to stop nursing until the infection is gone or until you have finished the course of antibiotics (do take the entire course). Continuing to nurse during mastitis will not harm your baby. The antibodies in your milk protect your baby from the infection, and the antibiotics prescribed for mastitis will not harm your baby. Frequent nursing, especially on the affected side, is essential to clear the duct. Mastitis tends to cause a mother's milk supply to drop, making her baby want to nurse almost constantly, which is the best treatment of all. The mastitis would certainly be aggravated if your breast became engorged, as it surely would if you abruptly weaned your baby. (Mastitis gone one step further is a breast abscess, or a localized collection of pus, that must be surgically drained.) As with plugged ducts, going to bed immediately with your baby to rest and nurse as much as possible will help you to overcome mastitis quickly and prevent it from returning.

Occasionally a baby is reluctant to nurse on an infected breast. If this is the case with your baby, offer the affected breast first when he is very hungry, asleep, or very sleepy. Try different nursing positions, or nurse him while walking or swaying. Mastitis can also make the areola hard, and difficult for the baby to grasp. To soften the areola, soak the area with a hot compress and gently express a little milk before you nurse. You may need to pump the affected breast while continuing to nurse the baby from it as much as possible (a baby can withdraw milk more effectively than a pump can).

Understanding how and why plugged ducts develop in the first place will help prevent them. They tend to occur when a feeding is missed, nursing is irregular, or the breasts are incompletely drained. Sometimes a woman takes great care to rest a lot and nurse often during the first few weeks at home, but then, when she feels ready to get out of the house and do more things, she does them with a vengeance, spending all day out and about. Not only does she nurse a little less than the day before, but she may tire herself out as well. (She may also wear a bag with a shoulder strap all day, as she gets her errands done, which could contribute to plugged ducts.) And the next morning she wakes up with a sore breast and, perhaps, a fever.

Ease back into your slate of activities gradually, keeping track of how often you're putting the baby to the breast. Anything that causes you to nurse less frequently can leave you dealing with a plugged duct. This can include your baby's sleeping for a longer stretch at night, introducing supplementary bottles, using a pacifier, or the hullabaloo surrounding holidays and house guests.

Incorrect positioning and poor latch-on and sucking, which so often cause sore nipples, can also lead to plugged ducts, by preventing your milk from flowing freely. If you suspect any one of these could be the cause of your plugged ducts or mastitis, call a lactation consultant or a La Leche League leader for one-on-one assistance. You want to be sure that your baby is draining at least one breast completely at each feeding.

Plugs can also be caused by anything that restricts the flow of milk in your breasts, including wearing an ill-fitting bra, carrying a heavy purse or diaper bag on your shoulder, wearing a backpack with shoulder straps, or carrying the baby in a front pack or in any manner that puts pressure on your breasts. Avoid wearing underwire bras, and go braless as much as possible, or at least switch to a bra with a larger cup and band size than you wore before pregnancy. Sleeping on your abdomen may also cause a plug.

Stress and fatigue can lead to plugged ducts, too. And since your resistance to infection is lower when you are under stress, any plugged duct you get while you are feeling stressed or exhausted is more likely to lead to an infection.

For mothers who do not plan to return to work, plugged ducts and mastitis are generally a thing of the past by the third month. Working mothers, however, may find themselves dealing with them all over again, or for the very first time, during their first weeks back at work. The causes are the same: an abrupt decrease in nursing frequency, incomplete emptying of the breasts, restrictive clothing, and stress or fatigue. Again, being aware of the causes will enable you to rid yourself of plugged ducts and mastitis in short order.

Mastitis will recur if it hasn't fully cleared up from the first time around, and it sometimes becomes a chronic problem. If you take antibiotics, be sure to finish the prescription and get extra rest for a good two weeks afterward.

If you have one bout of plugged ducts or mastitis after another, consider these questions:

◆ Are you getting enough fluids? Whether you are plagued by plugs or not, as a nursing mother you should be drinking a lot. Some women keep a liter water bottle with them at all times.

◆ Is your diet high in saturated fat? Some mothers say that limiting fat intake—even just switching from whole to skim milk—has dramatically helped them with recurrent plugged ducts.

◆ Are you using too much or too little salt? Excessive salt intake and chronic salt deficiency can both contribute to recurring mastitis.

◆ Was the right antibiotic prescribed at the right dose? Lactation consultants recommend a 10- to 15-day course of Keflex or dicloxacillin for mastitis.

Once identified, all potential causes of mastitis can be eliminated.

Carrying Your Baby

Answering a newborn's needs all day long can be inconvenient if not exhausting. What do you do if your baby cries every time you put him down? How do you brush your teeth or wash your hands? How do you take a shower or get yourself some lunch? How do you get anything done at all? In societies where women's domestic activities are essential to the survival of their families and, indeed, their communities, work does not cease when a baby is born. How do they do it? These working mothers wear their babies in slings or wrapped on their hips or their backs. Their hands are free to do the things that need to be done, while their babies are usually peaceful, contented companions.

In one study, babies who were carried most of the day cried 43 percent less than others. Why is a baby who is carried so much more content than one who is not? Babies born today are just the same as babies born thousands of years ago, long before carriages, cribs, and bouncy seats. They represent our three-million-year-old mammalian heritage unaltered. Humans are not birds or alligators who leave their babies in nests while they forage for food. Nor are we like hunting mammals, who leave their young in hidden lairs and return to nurse at widely spaced intervals. We are a "carrying" species, like apes and certain other mammals who keep our young with us while we work, eat, and sleep. We need to keep our babies close so we can nurse them often because our milk is low in fat compared with the milk of many other mammals. This is why a baby is born with a well-developed grasping reflex; it is intended to help him to hold on to his mother's body or hair. Like the sucking reflex, the grasping reflex is fully operational at birth because it was essential for our ancestors' survival.

The baby who is carried simply feels *right*. Infants crave motion. Ethologist Irenaus Eibl-Eibesfeldt observes that "mothers fondle their children in all cultures, lift them up or rock them in slumber. The rocking, jostling, and lifting of infants, which mothers enjoy doing so much, accommodates the infantile need for vestibular stimulation. An excited infant can be calmed by rocking it. Vestibular stimuli communicate to the infant that he is not alone."

> 66 As a fetus grows in the womb, surrounded by amniotic fluid, it feels liquid warmth, the heartbeat, the inner surf of the mother, and floats in a wonderful hammock that rocks gently as she walks. Birth must be a rude shock after such serenity, and a mother recreates the comfort of the womb in various ways (swaddling, cradling, pressing the baby against the left side of her body where her heart is). 99
>
> —DIANE ACKERMAN

The baby who is carried spends his days much as he did in the womb. The familiar role of his mother's stride, her soothing voice, and her heartbeat are all still constant. Carrying your baby allows him to spend these early months in a sort of fourth trimester, a comfortable transition to life on the outside.

Being carried prepares your baby for his future as an independent being as well as reminding him of his recent past. He can make eye contact with everyone around. Although he can sleep or nurse whenever he needs to, when he is alert he is a part of his mother's world, watching everything and joining in as soon as he is able. Said one mother, after carrying her four-month-old in a sling for the first time while cooking dinner, "The fun thing was how interested he was in everything I was doing. When I turned on the kitchen faucet he would reach for the water. When I opened the refrigerator, he peered inside. He watched fascinated as I cut veggies."

Carrying your baby won't make him clingy and unable to separate from you as he grows. Babies who are allowed to grow toward independence at their own pace are likely to achieve it earlier and more solidly than if they are hurried toward it. Among the Yequana Indians of South America, who carried their babies until they climbed down and crawled away, Jean Liedloff found the children precociously and astonishingly self-reliant. But exactly when your baby is ready to spend more time out of your arms will depend on his temperament. A baby born with a high need for tactile stimulation may prefer to be in a sling or pack until he starts to crawl, or even longer. A different baby may feel quite ready at three months to lie on a blanket watching a shaft of sunlight while you make breakfast.

When you are out and about, a sling, wrap, pack, or pouch gives you far more mobility than a stroller, which turns every door, stair, and narrow space into an obstacle to negotiate or avoid. A wearable cloth carrier also keeps your hands free to cook, write, sow seeds, pick up the phone, open the mail, or hold the hand of another child. By carrying your baby as mothers always have, you can meet your baby's needs and continue with all the activities of daily life at the same time.

Most importantly, carrying your baby vastly increases the amount of daily contact between the two of you. When you do return to work, the extended contact provided by carrying your baby during the hours you are at home will offset the effects of your daily separations. Indeed, frequent physical contact and interaction with your baby boosts your body's production of prolactin, the mothering hormone.

Fathers report that they, too, enjoy carrying their babies in slings and packs. The close physical contact gives a father and his baby a deep familiarity with the sound and scent and motions of the other. They will *know* each other far more than the father and baby who spend half an hour visiting a couple of times a day.

You can make or buy a sling or baby pack in any of numerous styles. Frontpacks are useful with small babies. Some models allow the baby to face forward so she can look out at the world. Most backpacks are best suited for older babies. They tend to put less strain on the shoulders and neck than frontpacks do, and they are safer to use while cooking in the kitchen.

A sling that drapes across your shoulder and around the opposite hip snuggles your baby—head, arms, legs, and all—in much the same comforting way the womb or a well-wrapped blanket does. A sling is also a cinch to take on and off; you don't need someone else's help to buckle it or to put the baby in. A sling also allows you to nurse discreetly in public; who can tell if the baby is sleeping or nursing when all one can see is the sling? Best of all, say mothers, is that if your baby falls asleep in the sling you can lay her down without waking her up simply by leaning over and sliding yourself backward out of the sling. She'll stay just as blissfully snuggled in the sling as she was when she first fell asleep. A sling can be used from birth to about three years (35 to 40 pounds)—much longer than a frontpack. Not only is a sling more comfortable and versatile for a growing baby than a frontpack, but it will be far more comfortable for you as time goes by, because it places the weight of your baby on your hips rather than on your shoulders.

A sling can feel awkward at first, but in time it will be easier to use than a frontpack or backpack. You may want to practice with a stuffed animal or doll before putting your baby in the sling. But do help your baby become accustomed to the sling as early as possible.

Most commercially available slings have a padded square to rest on your shoulder and a ring and pull-tab for adjusting the length of the sling. (Some parents prefer the non-adjustable styles, as they require less fussing with length.) They can be bought in maternity stores or on numerous online sites for baby and nursing supplies. You can also make your own sling out of a wide strip of sturdy fabric 1½ yards long; tie a strong knot at your shoulder.

To carry your baby in a sling—

◆ Lift it over your head, and place the padded square (or knot) on the edge of your left shoulder (if you are right handed). The ring and pull-tab on a commercially made sling should be in front of your shoulder. The sling should now hang across your body.

◆ Fluff out the fabric.

◆ Balance your baby on your right shoulder (the one without the ring or knot), and guide his feet into the sling. If your baby is a newborn, he should be fully swaddled in the fabric.

◆ If your baby is very small, you might fold a thin baby blanket or cloth diaper into a square, and tuck it under his head and shoulders for a little additional support.

◆ Pull up 3 to 5 inches of the fabric between your abdomen and the baby to secure him within both sides of the sling.

◆ To cinch up a commercially made sling, lift the baby's weight with one hand, and pull on the tab with the other hand.

◆ Walk with a little jiggle and pat the baby's bottom a bit to settle him in the sling.

Your baby will probably be happiest if you lay him in the sling with his head to your left. Mothers tend to carry their children on the left side (the side on which the sling is on your shoulder). Look at paintings and sculptures created through the centuries, and you will see that this has always been true the world over. This phenomenon has been thought to be due to the prevalence of right-handedness, since carrying the baby on the left frees the mother's right arm and hand. But left-handed mothers also tend to carry their babies on the left side.

Researchers have observed that newborns, when gently held facing forward, display clear preferences for turning their heads to one side or the other. About two-thirds of babies turn their heads to the right. (When they are held on the mother's left side, then, they turn to face her breast to hear the beat of her heart.) The other third, however, tend to turn to the left—and, researchers have found, their mothers tend to carry them on the *right.* You may already be carrying your baby on the side that reflects her innate preference. If your baby turns her head to the left and you tend to carry her on the right, put the sling's strap on your right shoulder.

When they are three or four months old, many babies like to sit up and look out at the world. This is when you might let your baby's legs dangle out at the front of the sling. Make sure the batting on the lower edge of a commercially made sling fully supports her knees and bottom. Or you can turn the baby around to sit cross-legged, so she faces the oncoming world. This position, as one mother says, is "very exciting for babies and little old ladies in the supermarket." As your baby gains control of her head, she will want to sit up in the sling more and more, straddling your hips with her legs, her bottom supported by the sling. With practice you will find that you can carry your baby on your back in the sling, which is especially useful when chopping vegetables in the kitchen or working at the computer.

Don't give up on the sling if your baby fusses at first; keep using it for a few days to let both of you grow accustomed to it. As with nursing, once you get the hang of a sling you will be able to use it anywhere, anytime.

If you aren't enjoying using a sling or baby pack, or your baby isn't, remember that carrying your baby, like breastfeeding, is just one of the tools of attachment in our human heritage. You don't need to carry your baby every second of every day to ensure that you and he develop a strong and harmonious bond. But if you find yourself hesitating to pick up your baby when he cries, or if someone tells you that "you're spoiling that baby by carrying him so much," remember that babies have always been picked up when they fuss and carried about by their mothers. Babies are still as they have always been; it is only adults and the cultures we compose that have changed.

Where Will Your Baby Sleep?

Sleepless nights are a hallmark of the newborn period. Your baby's admirers quickly follow "How old is she?" and "How much does she weigh?" with "Is she sleeping through the night yet?" Getting your baby to sleep through the night (whatever that means) is requisite to being a "good mother" (whatever *that* means). Mothers who are planning their return to work may feel desperate to ensure full nights of sleep as soon as possible. Their urgency may be due to a culture that reveres unbroken sleep and independent babies as much as their wish to be ready for work.

There are as many schools of thought on how to get babies to sleep all night as there are on the proper feeding of babies. One especially popular technique is to let the baby cry in her crib for increasingly long periods of time each night. Within a week, many babies trained in this way don't cry at night anymore. Proponents say the babies have learned to go to sleep on their own. They have become conditioned to being laid in their cribs, rather than being rocked or nursed, as a signal to go to sleep. Opponents of the method say the babies have learned that, no matter how much they cry, their wails won't be answered. They have reached a state of "learned helplessness." To new and tired parents, the two arguments may seem equally convincing.

Richard Ferber, the researcher and doctor who developed the method of teaching a baby to sleep over a period of days or weeks, admits that the technique "doesn't work for everyone." He adds that the alternative approach, co-sleeping, has "plenty of examples . . . where it works out just fine. My feeling now is that children can sleep with or without their parents. What's really important is that the parents work out what they want to do."

Many parents work out what they want to do by looking at the ways in which babies are cared for in most of the world. To these parents the Western taboo against letting babies sleep in their parents' beds doesn't make any sense. They discover that when they bring their babies into their own beds to sleep, everyone sleeps better. A new father admits with some amazement, "We didn't start out with a family bed. In fact, we were rather adamant that our son sleep in his own crib. But after weeks of getting up for feedings or getting up to check on the baby or getting up because the monitor was crackling, we decided to try having him sleep with us full time. It worked great! We got *more* sleep and our son seemed to sleep better, and to be more secure, too."

Despite the modern pronouncements against co-sleeping, in most societies babies sleep with their mothers. The United States is nearly unique, in fact, in its practice of discouraging babies from sleeping with their mothers. (Even other industrialized nations, including the United Kingdom, Australia, and New Zealand, are less zealous about keeping babies out of their mothers' beds.) In her book *Our Babies, Ourselves*, anthropologist Meredith Small cites a study of 186 non-industrial societies; in none of them do babies sleep in a separate place before they are at least a year old. In another study of 172 societies, all infants were found to do some co-sleeping at night.

It should be no surprise that breastfeeding is the cultural norm in these societies as well. Nursing a baby has a way of leading to nursing lying down, which tends to lead to nursing while sleeping, which is co-sleeping. As John Seabrook writes, "Co-sleeping is like the fine print at the bottom of the breastfeeding contract." In the evening, finishing a full meal at the breast, babies fall asleep mid-suckle. It's easy, then, to put them down in their cribs to sleep soundly while you eat your dinner and head to bed yourself. A little baby, however, is likely to request another meal around 11:00 P.M., and another between 1:00 and 5:00 A.M. He may fall asleep at the breast again, and be put down again in his crib after each of these nursings. Knowing, however, that he's going to want to nurse again in a few short hours, a mother may skip the getting-up-and-putting-down process, and simply stay cuddled with the baby in her bed from one nursing to the next.

The effort to get babies to sleep alone at night has led to ways to get them to skip those nighttime meals. Putting baby cereal into bottles has been the advice of grandmothers and neighbors for decades to "help the baby sleep longer." While adding cereal has not been shown to increase the length of babies' sleep cycles (although it has been shown to increase the risk of Type 1 diabetes in babies with a family history of the disease), formula-fed babies do wake a little less at night, on average, than breastfed babies. The cow's milk curds formed in the stomach of a formula-fed baby are tougher and more difficult to digest than the small, soft, easily digested curds of breast milk. Formula-fed babies can go slightly longer between feedings (up to four hours), because they feel fuller longer.

Nature intends babies to nurse at night. A nursing mother's prolactin levels are highest between 1:00 A.M. and 5:00 A.M., and her milk has a higher fat content at night. Without nursing at night, her breasts will be overfull by morning, and this will reduce her overall milk production.

If a baby spends the night alone, he must wake fully when he is hungry, and cry long and loud enough to be heard by his sleeping mother. She too must wake fully, leave her bed and go to his room, pick him up, settle in a chair to nurse, then nurse him, rock him back to sleep, and ever so carefully place him back in his crib without waking him up. Then she returns to her bed. This process may be repeated every two or three hours through the night. (Imagine adding a trip to the kitchen to prepare a bottle of formula to all that nocturnal activity!)

Consider the difference if your baby sleeps within your reach, in your bed or in a "sidecar crib" attached to your bed. He begins to snuffle and make sucking motions in his sleep. You wake just enough to draw him close to your breast. He latches on and nurses without ever crying or waking completely. As he nurses, you fall back into a light sleep. When he is satiated, he falls back into a deep sleep. Neither of you has woken fully, and you both feel comforted because the other is near. Your mate sleeps soundly on the other side of the bed, usually unaware of your ministrations. (What about changing your baby's diaper? Unless he is really soaked and leaking, don't bother until morning.)

Proponents say that co-sleeping, like picking your baby up when he cries, teaches him trust. He knows that you are always there for him, that you will be there for him when he stumbles, and this knowledge frees him to grow toward independence. He forms a sense of what child psychologist Erik Erikson called "basic trust"; he can safely risk growing up.

Experienced working nursing mothers say the benefits are more immediate. Being near their babies at night gives them an additional eight to nine hours a day in which they are in close contact. Although they may not be fully conscious for much of the night, they are still in physical contact, interacting in the most subtle and harmonious way.

Keeping your baby near you at night also prepares you for the possibility of reverse-cycle feeding. Some babies whose mothers are away five or more hours a day tend to sleep more during the day than other babies and to stay awake, socialize, and nurse more in the evenings and at night. When Mom is not around, the baby saves his energy. But when reunited with Mom, the baby more than makes up for the hours apart. This is a lovely and touching adjustment, a tribute a baby pays to his beloved mother. Keeping your baby beside you at night makes it possible for you to accept this natural adjustment and still get the rest you need.

Allowing your baby to nurse at night will also maintain your milk supply while you are working. A baby who reverses his cycle of rest and activity may not drink all of the pumped breast milk Mom has left at the sitter's; he is getting most of the nourishment he needs during the time he is with his mother, and would rather wait for her to provide his meals, thank you very much. If you're nursing a lot at night, you may be able to give up pumping your milk sooner than otherwise.

The American Academy of Pediatrics (AAP) is concerned about a possible association between co-sleeping and Sudden Infant Death Syndrome (SIDS). Reviewing the results of multiple large-scale studies, the AAP concluded in 2005 that the risk of SIDS is slightly increased when babies sleep alone and also when they sleep on "a surface not designed for infant sleep" (including any mattress other than a crib mattress), but is reduced when babies sleep in the same room as their mothers. The data also suggest that the risk of SIDS is slightly reduced when babies are given pacifiers to suck on as they fall asleep. The AAP therefore recommended that babies sleep in cribs in their mother's rooms, but not in their beds, and that they be offered pacifiers at bedtime.

The response to the AAP's revised recommendations has been mixed, to say the least. Objections were raised by UNICEF and the World Health Organization, originators of the Baby-Friendly Hospital Initiative. (Hospitals are awarded "baby-friendly" status when standard procedures in maternity wards are brought into line with the breastfeeding guidelines developed by WHO and UNICEF. Baby-Friendly USA, the American branch of the initiative, is working toward "an American culture that values the enduring benefits of breastfeeding and human milk for mothers, babies, and society.") La Leche League, the international association for breastfeeding mothers, and the [American] Academy of Breastfeeding Medicine (ABM) also objected to the recommendations. Dr. Nancy Wight, then-president of the ABM, commented that the AAP statement "represents a truly astounding triumph of ethnocentric assumptions over common sense and medical research." Dr. Wight added, "There are many physician members of the AAP who do not agree with these recommendations." La Leche League declared that the AAP statement "causes confusion for parents and falls seriously short of being a useful and comprehensive policy."

In response to the AAP's recommendations, UNICEF and Britain's National Child Trust issued a joint statement in 2005 urging that parents "be given clear, accurate information on the risk factors of SIDS so that they can make their own decisions." The statement pointed out that breastfed babies are less likely to succumb to SIDS than formula-fed babies, and that supporting breastfeeding is therefore a powerful precaution to help babies sleep safely. The statement added, "There is evidence that mothers who breastfeed and share a bed with their babies are more likely to continue breastfeeding. As not breastfeeding is associated with increased short and long term health risks, we are worried that telling women not to co-sleep may reduce the duration of breastfeeding." Co-sleeping builds and maintains a mother's milk supply by encouraging regular and frequent feeding without sacrificing a mother's sleep. The UNICEF statement also pointed out that no study yet done on the safety of co-sleeping had controlled for known risk factors for SIDS—smoking, drug and alcohol use by parents, and inappropriate sleep surfaces such as sofas and waterbeds.

The AAP's endorsement of pacifier use stirred up more confusion and concern. As La Leche League pointed out, "The recommendations about pacifiers and co-sleeping reflect a lack of basic understanding about breastfeeding management. Pacifiers . . . are artificial substitutes for what the breast does naturally. Breastfed babies often nurse to sleep for naps and bedtime. The recommended pacifier usage could cause a reduction in milk supply due to reduced stimulation of the breasts and may affect breastfeeding duration." UNICEF pointed out that the data suggest that pacifiers may offer additional protection against SIDS, but only if they are used every night. If a baby is routinely given a pacifier as he falls asleep, but misses the occasional night, then the risk of SIDS is higher on the nights a pacifier is not used than if a pacifier were never used. Is it realistic, asks UNICEF, to expect that once a pacifier is used to help a baby fall asleep, it will continue to be used every night without fail?

The AAP recommendations don't explain why a pacifier provides some protection against SIDS, but the mechanism can be surmised. Pacifiers stimulate sucking, which comforts a baby and keeps the baby at a low level of arousal during sleep. This slight on-again-off-again arousal, suggests the research of Dr. James McKenna, director of the Mother-Baby Behavioral Sleep Laboratory at the University of Notre Dame, may prevent babies from falling so deeply asleep that their immature nervous systems cannot regulate breathing. What else stimulates steady sucking on and off during sleep? A mother's breast, when it is close by and available throughout the night.

Parents the world over sleep safely with their babies, and SIDS rarely occurs in societies where all babies sleep with their mothers. If you choose to bring your baby into your bed to nurse at night, do not smoke, use illicit or sedating drugs, or drink alcohol before bed. Sleep on a firm mattress, never on a waterbed, sofa, or other soft surface on which it would be difficult for the baby to lift his head and keep his nose clear for breathing. A baby is safest between a mother and her mate (who must also avoid smoking, drugs, and alcohol), so long as the baby's head and face are clear of pillows, sheets, and blankets. If a baby sleeps between his parents, move the parents' pillows away, toward the sides of the bed. Blankets and sheets can be pulled down in the center of the bed so that they do not cover the baby, who can be kept warm by a sleepsuit, a light baby blanket, and his parents' warmth. If a baby sleeps on the mother's side away from the middle of the bed, the bed must pressed up against the wall without any gap or potential for a gap through which the baby could fall. The ideal arrangement is a "sidecar crib" attached to the adult bed and open on one side to the mother's side of the bed. With one of these, the baby can sleep in his own space, yet he is within his mother's reach for nursing and cuddling. A bassinet or cradle by the side of the bed is another alternative to a crib in a separate room.

Once you let your baby into your bed or room, you may wonder, will he ever leave? Babies eventually wean themselves of their parents' bed and room just as they do of their mothers' milk, although you can hurry along the process, if you like. Some couples love waking up with a cuddly two-year-old; others move the baby into a bed of his own at around six months. Either way, when the transition is made gradually and tenderly, your baby will eventually learn to sleep securely in his own bed. (Snazzy new sheets printed with favorite cartoon characters or fire trucks have been known to work wonders with toddlers.) You may find that, long after your child has begun sleeping in his own bed, he still makes his way to yours when he needs you—when he has had a bad dream, when he is sick, or when he is feeling stressed by some events in his life. Again, seeking you out in the night is not a discipline problem; it is a measure of the depth of your attachment.

What about your privacy? Frankly, most of it was lost the moment your baby was born—and you are unlikely to get it back until your youngest child leaves home. But what little privacy you have can be found in places other than your bed. Many parents keep part of the night to themselves by rocking and nursing the baby to sleep at bedtime, putting him in the crib until he wakes, then bringing him into their bed when he wakes a few hours later.

Caring for Yourself

No matter how you care for your baby, you will find it hard going unless you care for yourself as well. In the first eight weeks following your baby's birth, take extra care to be sure that you are resting enough and eating well. Not only are you making tremendous emotional adjustments, but your body is nourishing another human being, besides recovering from the stress of giving birth and reverting to its prepregnant state. Getting too little rest at this time can lead to problems that can quickly snowball into a miserable situation that may include mastitis, breastfeeding failure, or depression. Obey the cardinal rule of the postpartum period: Sleep when the baby sleeps. Even a 20-minute catnap can do wonders for your well-being.

If you are standing, sit. If you are sitting, lie down. If you are lying down, sleep. These guidelines become imperatives if you have given birth by cesarean section.

Pay close attention to your nutritional needs during these postpartum weeks. Nursing mothers are usually thirsty and eager to drink copious amounts of fluids. Let your mate know that one of the most helpful things he can do for you while he is home is to be sure that you always have a large glass of water or juice next to you when you sit down to nurse. You may feel intensely thirsty the moment your milk lets down; in this way nature reminds you that you need fluids. (You needn't drown yourself in fluids, though. Just drink when you're thirsty.)

If you don't drink a lot of milk normally, don't feel as though you must drink it now. You don't need to drink cow's milk to make human milk. Cow's milk is a convenient source of necessary protein and calcium, but both nutrients can be found in a lot of other foods. Indeed, too much cow's milk in your diet may make your baby uncomfortable.

This is not the time to go on a weight-loss diet. Breastfeeding women generally lose the extra weight they put on in pregnancy without any special effort, as long as they eat sensibly. It is believed that a nursing mother of normal weight needs about 500 calories more each day than she did before pregnancy to cover the energy requirements of lactation. The sensible advice is to eat when you are hungry and not beyond satiation.

The quality of your breast milk does not depend on the quality of the food you eat; your milk-producing glands will draw on your body for any vitamins, minerals, or protein missing from your diet but needed for milk production. This tends to occur, however, only when a mother is truly malnourished. Although you now can eat more than you used to, this does not mean that you can fill up on "cheat foods" such as cake and sweet rolls. If you do, you won't lose weight, and you'll tend to feel tired and "used up." While you are breastfeeding, especially during the first weeks postpartum, you need extra protein and extra calcium. Tuck into well-balanced meals of beans, meat, chicken, cheese, eggs, or fish; fresh fruits and green or orange vegetables; and brown rice and other whole grains. A good diet does not need to be an expensive diet. Rice and beans are more nutritious and less costly than processed and packaged foods. Stock the refrigerator and cupboards with nourishing foods you can prepare quickly, especially ones high in protein. You're less likely to skimp, or to fill up on doughnuts, if something better is within easy reach. Oatmeal, hard-boiled eggs, nuts, canned tuna, baked or refried beans, and tofu all make nearly instant, nutritious snacks or meals. Your baby will be fine whatever you eat, but you will feel better if you eat good food during the first few weeks.

If your physician or midwife prescribed a multivitamin and iron supplement while you were pregnant, continue taking it as long as you are nursing. If you are not taking a multivitamin, you may want to take a daily B-complex supplement since a lack of B vitamins can cause depression and anxiety. Brewer's yeast, a natural source of B vitamins, iron, and protein, is very good for nursing mothers (another reason midwives recommended dark ale).

Although breastfeeding generally doesn't limit a mother's diet in any way, sometimes a young baby will fuss for a day or so after his mother has eaten a specific food. Common culprits are caffeine, cow's milk and dairy products, chocolate, onions, cabbage, broccoli, Brussels sprouts, cauliflower, beans, garlic, cinnamon, tomatoes, and citrus fruits. Many babies wouldn't mind a bit if their mothers made an entire meal of these foods. But if your baby is very fussy one day, suddenly refuses to nurse, has gas or diarrhea, or has a rash or redness around the anus, review your diet over the past 24 hours. You will want to rule out other possible causes, of course, but if you think something you ate is at fault, eliminate from your diet for two to three days any food you suspect. If your baby's troubles are caused by something in your diet, he is likely to fuss from two to eight hours after you have ingested it.

Simplification

You can create a more restful atmosphere in your home by simplifying your life wherever and whenever possible. The cliché that something worth doing is worth doing well just isn't true, at least not at this stage in your life. Right now, if something is barely worth doing, then barely do it. Review your housekeeping standards, and decide how much you can reduce your chores in ways that won't make a discernible difference (and even if it is discernible, who cares?). A few ways families have cut back include:

- ◆ Arrange for someone else to clean your home, or be satisfied with shortcut cleaning.

- ◆ Leave the breakfast dishes (all right, and the lunch and dinner dishes, too) soaking in the sink until you are good and ready to do them. Better yet, use paper plates.

- ◆ Make simple meals, and indulge in nutritious take-out food.

- ◆ Ask a friend or relative who likes to cook for a week's worth of meals that can be frozen, in place of a present for the baby.

- ◆ Use disposable diapers for the time being, or for good.

- ◆ Vacuum the middle of the room, but skip going under the sofa. (Or don't vacuum at all. Imagine that!)

- ◆ Leave socks and clean diapers in a basket to be retrieved as needed rather than sorting and putting them away.

- ◆ Unclutter your house so that you have less to clean; box up all those knickknacks for the next five years.

- ◆ Use an answering machine to screen phone calls.

- ◆ Say no as much as possible to requests and intrusions.

- ◆ Use a portable phone so you can answer the phone without getting up.

- ◆ Pay your bills online or by automatic transfer.

You may want to extend these simplification measures, and any others you devise, through the first year or more after you return to work. They are as helpful to working mothers as they are to mothers of newborns.

Enlisting Help from Your Partner

Somehow, when a woman becomes responsible for every need of her baby, she often becomes responsible for every need of her family. Perhaps your division of duties before the baby was born was completely egalitarian. Your partner cooked dinner; you mowed the lawn. You washed and dried the laundry; he folded it and put it away. But even the most modern and fair arrangements tend to become more traditional when a baby enters the equation.

To prevent being saddled with all the cooking, cleaning, and other jobs that your home life requires (or to unsaddle yourself), enlist your partner's help, and applaud his efforts. You are far more likely to get him to do what you need with praise than with criticism. And once he is doing the minimum you need (coming home in time to cook dinner, doing a few loads of laundry), he is more likely to take on additional responsibilities if he knows that you are pleased with his efforts so far.

Keep in mind that your partner's idea of an adequate meal or a clean room may differ from yours. The continual inadequacy of men's housework can be infuriating to women; as a result, many men feel that there is no point in offering to do things, since their wives always get mad and tell them they've done it wrong. If you praise your partner's efforts, these attempts are more likely to improve and become proud and established skills. Help from him with the household now will enable you to focus on learning to breastfeed and getting to know your baby. His help when you return to work may make the difference between successfully blending work and home life or becoming utterly exhausted by your dual roles. In 1989, Arlie Hochschild, a sociologist, measured the time women and men spend in housework and child care in addition to their paid work, and discovered that "women worked roughly fifteen hours longer each week than men. Over a year, they worked an extra month of twenty-four hour days." As Hochschild observed in her book *The Second Shift*, "Just as there is a wage gap between men and women in the workplace, there is a 'leisure gap' between them at home. Most women work one shift at the office or factory and a 'second shift' at home."

In the years since her book brought this gap to light, change has been slow to come. Statistically, more men are doing a significant share of the work at home, but they're still a minority. Paula Malone, an economist at the University of Michigan, has seen a shift, but not a large one. "Despite a slight reallocation of housework activities from wives to husbands in recent years, most of the housework as well as the care of children within the home is still primarily the re-sponsibility of the woman," she says. "Wives are still primarily doing 'women's work,' such as meals, dishes, cleaning, shopping and laun-dry, whereas men are engaged in the traditional male tasks, such as yard work, home maintenance and auto repair." Her research reveals another interesting fact: While the number of hours they spend on housework does not affect the wages of men of any age, the income of young women (ages 20 to 34) and middle-aged women (ages 35 to 49) is reduced by the amount of housework they do.

Feeling Blue and Finding Support

New motherhood can jostle your emotional life whether you plan to return to work or not. Mood swings, sudden inexplicable tears, and feeling vulnerable and overwhelmed are common during the first six weeks. They're known as the baby blues, and a mother's susceptibil-ity to them generally peaks at the third day after birth (about when the milk comes in) and subsides about two to three weeks after birth. Maybe we tend to feel rocky during these early weeks because we so often give birth and care for our newborns in biologically bizarre cir-cumstances—alone or among strangers, and without experienced mothers to guide us. Shifting hormone levels and fatigue also play a role, but if you're lacking emotional support you need to seek some out. Attend a La Leche League meeting or a reunion of your childbirth class. Sign up for a mother-baby exercise class to meet other new mothers. Check the bulletin boards at your public library and church for notices of new-mothers' groups forming, or form one yourself. Seek out especially other nursing mothers who plan to return to work, and talk with mothers at your workplace who were supportive during your pregnancy. Sharing your concerns with other parents is more than practical; it is sustenance for your soul. As someone who has devoted much of her time and energy to work, you may now need to build a network of home- and child-focused friends. Doing so does not mean you are losing your old life and friends; you are only expanding your circle to include people who can share this new stage in your life. The friends you make through your children will be the ones who will be there for you when you desperately need a babysitter or a ride to the emergency room. They will be your source of recommendations for a doctor, dentist, school, or place to find used ice skates.

If you have a computer and Internet access, seek out other parents in cyberspace. You can find online forums on every conceivable subject related to parenting: newborns, breastfeeding, working mothers, attachment parenting, single mothers, egalitarian parenting, executive mothers, and more. The messages shared in these online groups make fascinating reading. Every problem you are facing or might face in the future is likely to be discussed by participants. Ask for advice on sore nipples, sleepless nights, finding daycare, or choosing a breast pump, and you are likely to receive a dozen helpful and empathetic responses from parents who have been in your precise situation. One mother echoed many when she wrote, "Thank goodness for all of you. I don't know how I would have gotten through the last few weeks without your help." You may find Web sites helpful, too; especially helpful sites for parents and working women are listed in the Resources section (pages 217-18).

Simple activities can dramatically lift your mood as well. For example—

◆ Take a daily walk in the afternoon sun with the baby tucked in a sling or frontpack. The fresh air and exercise will do you both good.

◆ Walk to a nearby playground; you'll probably find other parents to commiserate and rejoice with.

◆ Go downtown or to a mall just to window-shop and people-watch.

◆ If you feel like crying, let your tears flow. The shower is a great place to sob unselfconsciously. Cry out loud right along with your baby; you're certain to feel better when you are done.

◆ Buy a new outfit that is comfortable, easy to nurse in, and pretty, too.

◆ Take a long bath while your mate holds the baby, or take a bath with your baby.

◆ Rent a funny movie to watch while you are nursing.

◆ Call someone who makes you laugh.

◆ While you nurse, read *Operating Instructions,* Anne Lamott's hilarious and insightful memoir of her son's first year. If you can't manage a full-length book right now, try *A Teeny Tiny Baby*, Amy Schwartz's brilliant, tender, and very funny picture book for children.

If your baby blues seem more than mild—if you feel so sad that you are nearly immobilized—you may be experiencing postpartum depression. True postpartum depression usually begins three weeks to five months after birth. Professional help is essential; talk to your doctor or your baby's pediatrician about finding expert help now. Please note that the AAP has just issued a policy based on the results of a new study advising pediatricians to screen new mothers for postpartum depression, as they often see the moms more than do the mother's own doctors.

When you feel overwhelmed and anxious, remember that your feelings are normal. They do not mean that you are better suited to your life at work than to life as a mother. If you have always placed a priority on feeling in charge, try to put aside that need during these weeks as you open yourself up to motherhood. You may be considering cutting short your maternity leave or hiring a baby nurse in an attempt to regain control and return your life to normality, but doing so would only slow your adjustment to motherhood and put a distance between you and your baby. The first few weeks on any new job feel chaotic and overwhelming; motherhood is no different.

Although right now this lifetime commitment you've made fills every minute of every day, it won't always be so. Your baby will not always want to nurse every two hours, and you will not always be bleary-eyed and in your pajamas. You will figure out not only how to accomplish a shower and lunch in the same day, but how to get your baby and yourself dressed and out the door by 8:00 A.M. In fact, with time, the organizational and coping skills you gain as a mother will reach astonishing heights—and you are likely to find yourself applying them to your professional work as well. As Katherine Ellison explains in *The Mommy Brain: How Motherhood Makes Us Smarter,* the work of nurturing our babies, as well as the hormones released during the nurturing, can literally reshape our brains, making them more flexible and complex, improving our ability to accomplish any task.

Meanwhile, allow nursing to become your source of peace and release, providing tranquil departures from the clamoring demands of the world. And your baby, your partner in a mutually rewarding relationship, will serve as your ally in blending your many roles into one harmonious whole.

five

PREPARING TO GO
BACK TO WORK

WHETHER YOUR EARLIEST WEEKS as a mother are smooth or rough, a day will certainly come when everything suddenly seems a little easier. You've learned a lot about your baby by the end of the first four to six weeks. You know when she is hungry, you can tell when she needs to sleep, you have a repertoire of ways to comfort her. If you go to the supermarket without her, you miss her within twenty minutes and hurry to get home again. You have left the initial learning period behind and have entered the reward period, when breastfeeding and caring for your baby are much less perplexing and even a lot of fun.

Whereas mothers who plan to stay home indefinitely can relax at this point and thoroughly enjoy their babies, your mind may be on the rapidly approaching day when you will return to work. You've entered a stage that is unique to working mothers.

In some ways this period feels like those last weeks of pregnancy; it is marked by anticipation, anxiety, and the sense that you don't really know what's waiting for you just around the corner.

Mothers planning to go back to work experience a wide range of emotions at this time. Much depends on how you feel about your work. Do you love it? If so, you may be eager to be back at it, or you may feel a bittersweet tug in two directions. Do you work just for the money and benefits, and would you quit if you could? If so, you may be feeling especially stressed at this time. Whether you are grief-stricken or raring to go, the intensity of your feelings in this period is entirely normal. You've hit the rapids, the whitecaps and whirlpools where two rivers converge in the lives of women in the twenty-first century. There are no time-honored traditions to guide us here; each of us finds her own way through these waters.

Maybe you feel comfortable with your decision to work but worry about the logistics. You may still find it a challenge to get yourself and your baby out of the house and to the supermarket by noon. How will you get the baby to daycare and yourself to work by nine o'clock every morning? How will you attend that out-of-town sales conference in two months or work a ten-hour shift without weaning your baby? The questions hover like biting flies.

Take this first year of motherhood one day at a time. Know that your abilities will expand with the demands you put upon them—not infinitely, but further than you might ever have thought possible. Try to brush away worrying questions for now. One of the lessons of motherhood is that you needn't plan everything in fixed detail, because your plans are likely to be disrupted anyway. Trust that you will figure out the right thing to do when you need to do it. Know that solutions will evolve, that you will find answers when you need them. Mothering can teach you to ride life instead of directing it, to be open to unexpected opportunities and ready for sudden turns in the road. You will learn to respond to the rest of your life as spontaneously and intuitively as you do to your baby's cues and needs.

Whether you are looking forward to going back to your job or dreading it, know that you have already put into place the element most important to your success in blending your working life and your home life: your attachment to your baby. A strong attachment will prevent the hours you spend apart from disturbing the harmony of your relationship and interfering with the development of your nurturing skills. Continue to care for your baby as you began, using the tools in your parenting toolbox: breastfeeding the baby and responding quickly to her cues, and carrying her about and keeping her near you at night, if these work for you. These ancient ways of mothering can help you ensure that you and your baby will stay in tune despite your daily separations and the distractions of work. Breastfeeding in particular will not only keep you and your baby close, but it will supply you with constant, reassuring evidence of your unique place at the center of your baby's world.

Reconnecting with the Outside World

Since you gave birth, you may have put aside all thought of the world beyond the baby in your arms. Once you may not have believed that your world could become so contracted; now it may be hard to imagine leaving the cozy cocoon of your home. If so, your first task may be to restretch your boundaries so that you feel comfortable and confident in the outside world. You can begin simply by nursing in new places around your home or while you are doing something else—working at the computer, or talking on the phone. Try nursing at a friend's house. Move on to nursing in a restaurant or in a changing room at a clothing shop. When you're really comfortable, try a park bench.

Nursing in public may be a hurdle for you—or it may not. As one mother admits, "Shyness is not my strong point right now." Either way, you'll want to learn how to nurse discreetly so that you can nurse wherever you wish without anxiety, no matter the circumstances. Practice at home until you can put your baby to the breast without fumbling. When you are ready to nurse outside your home, wear a large, loose T-shirt or blouse to cover you well and give you plenty of room to maneuver; lift the shirt to nurse, or unbutton it from the bottom. Wearing a sweater or a jacket over your shirt will cover your sides as you lift up your shirt. Or treat yourself to some clothes especially designed for nursing mothers, with buttoned flaps and hidden slits that allow you to nurse both discreetly and fashionably (see Resources, page 217). For more privacy, a shawl or a baby blanket draped across your shoulder can form a tent over your baby as you nurse.

Wearing your baby in a sling can make discreet nursing infinitely easier. One particularly adept mother found that by nursing her four-week-old in a sling she could keep both her hands free to run the white-elephant booth at her four-year-old's nursery school. Her blouse had a small flap that opened for nursing, so she didn't have to pull it up or unbutton it. No one buying a cast-off asparagus steamer or shoe rack ever knew that her baby was doing something other than sleeping.

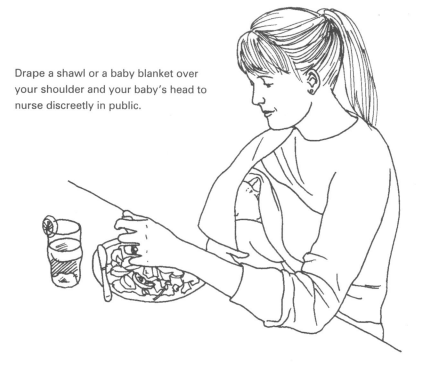

Drape a shawl or a baby blanket over your shoulder and your baby's head to nurse discreetly in public.

Try not to feel embarrassed if people notice that you're breastfeeding in public. Nursing openly and proudly reminds people that breasts are first and foremost for feeding babies, and helps our society to become a more welcoming place for mothers and babies.

Right now, of course, your goal is not to change the world, but to return to it along with your baby. Leaving the baby at home while you venture forth might initiate a habit of dividing your life into separate, independent spheres—baby here, work there, while you desperately race back and forth. The result could be utter exhaustion for you and, possibly, a developing distance between you and your baby. Your baby does not want to keep you at home; he simply wants to be with you wherever you go.

Nursing while doing other things at home helps to blend the spheres of your life. When you and your baby are a proficient breastfeeding couple, you may find that you can write letters, work at the computer, or do any number of things while nursing. An ability to nurse while doing desk work or talking on the telephone, in particular, may be key to your success in blending working and mothering in the coming year.

Reconnecting with Your Workplace

If you are taking two to three months off, you may wish to increase communication with your workplace in the second half of your maternity leave. Consider carefully if, when, and how you'll go about this. If you think that talking with your colleagues and perhaps even bringing some work home will make you feel like yourself again, exercise caution. Be certain that you're not hurrying back to work to escape the bewildering demands of your baby. You could end up circumventing motherhood rather than integrating it into your identity—and the result would be a distance between you and your child. Focus on becoming in tune with your baby and comfortable in your role as his mother. Perhaps you should consider *extending* rather than shortening your maternity leave (see Extending Your Maternity Leave, page 128).

If you feel comfortable and confident in your new role as mother, however, reconnecting with work before the end of your maternity leave might benefit you and your baby in the long run. One mother, a sales representative for a publishing company, brought her four-week-old baby into the office to show him off to her colleagues. While there, she casually let her department manager know that she might have time to do some work at home. She left with a stack of paperwork and a mountain of goodwill. As her baby was settling into a pattern of taking a two-hour morning nap and another in the late afternoon, she managed to get quite a lot of the work done, and, because she hadn't made any promises, she didn't worry about the rest. To show her dedication, she called in a couple of times with questions and comments and even attended a meeting at the office.

Her decision to join the meeting in the sixth week of her maternity leave was especially well considered. She volunteered to come, explaining that her participation would help keep her up to speed while she was on leave. Because all had gone well when she'd brought in the baby for a visit, she brought him along to the meeting as well. "I considered asking permission first," she says, "but I thought they might say no because they'd assume that my baby would disrupt the meeting. I knew he wouldn't and wanted to prove it." She showed up, baby in the sling and notebook in her hand, as if she never imagined his presence would be a problem. If any of her colleagues were surprised, they concealed their reaction. Sitting down at the conference table with her sleeping baby snugly out of sight in the sling, the sales rep turned her attention to the business at hand. The others, taking their cue from her, did the same. When the baby stirred and began to wake at one point, she calmly stood and walked around the room to settle him back to sleep, continuing to participate in the discussion as she did so. The meeting ended shortly thereafter, and she found a private office in which to nurse the baby before heading home.

Asked if she would have nursed the baby, if necessary, during such a meeting, she says, "It depends. If just the people I work closely with were there, I might have nursed discreetly in the room. If others were there with whom I have more formal relationships, and the baby couldn't be satisfied for the time being by sucking on my finger, I might have excused myself to nurse him for five or ten minutes somewhere else—just as someone else might have excused himself to take an important phone call. But I made sure that we nursed just before going to the meeting. I also asked that the meeting be scheduled during the late morning, when I knew he was likely to be sleeping."

This confident, flexible woman demonstrated to her colleagues that she was still a full member of their team without ever camouflaging her new role as a mother. She refused to accept the notion that the mere presence of her baby would diminish her professionalism. Knowing that a fussing, unhappy baby would indeed interrupt the meeting and prevent everyone from getting as much work done as they had planned, she met her baby's needs before they became disruptive demands, while keeping her focus on the meeting. By the end of the meeting all present had revised their attitude about children in the office—and patted themselves on the back for being such an open-minded, progressive company.

Best yet, however, was that when this mother approached her manager about the possibility of working four days a week for the first three months after she returned, her request was granted because she had accomplished so much work during her maternity leave. That four-day week eventually evolved to a five-day week with two of those days spent working at home. Her manager agreed to the latter as a permanent arrangement because he had full confidence that the presence of her child would not stop this employee from getting her work done.

And he was right. She was able to blend her dual roles into one because her work and her mothering did not conflict with each other. Her baby rarely made it impossible for her to work because she made meeting both his physical and emotional needs her first priority—and because she scheduled her work around the times when she knew his needs would be high. Her work rarely disrupted her life as a mother because she refused to stop being a mother while she swam in "professional" waters.

Anyone who has ever attended a La Leche League (LLL) conference has seen many mothers, both lactation professionals and lay leaders, accomplishing the same seamless blending of mothering and other activities. At any regional or national LLL conference, a hundred or more parents spend two to three days in a hotel attending seminars, workshops, and keynote luncheons—just as stockbrokers, computer scientists, and widget salesmen do at their conventions. The difference is that LLL conventions are also attended by about 200 children under the age of five. Two- and three-year-olds may run in a circle in the back of a meeting room; a mother with a fussy two-month-old may leave a seminar briefly to comfort her crying baby in the hallway, knowing that someone will catch her up on what she is missing. The adults' tolerance for the children's presence and normal behavior, and their willingness to assist one another, allow them to work productively while meeting their children's needs. And because these needs are met, the children rarely become disruptive.

This doesn't mean that you should launch a campaign to do away with daycare and bring everyone's children into your workplace. But neither should you assume that children and work simply do not mix. Consider ways that you might possibly blend work and mothering. If you find yourself immediately dismissing any such possibilities, examine your own assumptions. Bringing your child to work may not be best for either of you, but there may be other ways that you can blend the two sides of your life. The last sections of this chapter may give you some ideas.

Finding Substitute Care for Your Baby

Returning to work will be infinitely easier if you have found someone you trust to care for your baby while you are gone. Unfortunately, daycare—and the prospect of searching for it—has become the bogeyman of working parents. The media gleefully tell daycare horror stories without ever mentioning the happy relationships that exist between so many families and their babysitters, nannies, and daycare providers. Too often, daycare is considered a modern invention, a risky experiment with young lives and family structures.

In fact, daycare is nothing new and, as recent research reveals, usually beneficial. In most traditional societies, as soon as a child can walk she spends much of her day in a play group of children of mixed ages. She is cared for by a babysitter, usually an older girl who has grown up as a member of the play group herself. Eibl-Eibesfeldt, the ethologist, observes how a child develops in such a setting: The baby watches the group, imitates the older children, and plays simple games with the babysitter. At about age three, the child joins the play directly. "It is in such play groups that children are truly raised," says Eibl-Eibesfeldt.

Group care for children is not only nearly universal in human society, but it offers significant benefits to its participants. The children learn early on that they are a part of a larger community—and they become committed to the well-being of that community right from the beginning. Their social skills are taught and polished by other children, who will be their peer group for life. Each child becomes well-versed in the rich culture of childhood, learning its games and songs and etiquette and bequeathing this culture to children who follow her. As the younger children watch and learn from the older ones, the older ones practice their nurturing skills and begin their climb toward responsible adulthood. Babies are picked up, talked to, cuddled, and played with by children of all ages and by the adults around them. These children develop strong relationships with numerous adults and peers, to everyone's pleasure and benefit.

In our society, unfortunately, daycare is not always so safe, loving, and appropriately educational. A baby left from dawn to dusk in a large daycare center with an ever-changing cast of caregivers is not going to benefit from the experience. But when daycare is closer to the traditional model, research has shown, children thrive. They receive the social and intellectual stimulation that children have enjoyed through time.

But how, you may wonder, will regular substitute care affect your baby's relationship with you? What if a daycare provider is so wonderful that she and the baby become very close? Can this intimate relationship weaken the mother-infant bond? Again, research studies (and human history) say no. A child can form a loving attachment to several other adults while maintaining a primary attachment to his mother and father.

A long-term study funded by the National Institute of Child Health and Human Development is following 1,200 children from birth through the first grade and beyond to determine the effects of daycare on their psychological and cognitive development and physical health. At one, six, and fifteen months, daycare appears to have *no effect* on the children's attachment to their mothers, "regardless of the quality of the care, the age when the child entered it, or the type of care—whether provided by a father, a grandparent, another family or a daycare center."

The latest report has a critical caveat, however. It is this: "Child care can make a bad situation worse. If a mother is insensitive to a child's needs, having the child in daycare will further weaken the attachment between the two." In other words, even high-quality daycare can harm your child's development if your attachment is insecure. Continuing to breastfeed and to draw on the other attachment-promoting tools in your parenting toolbox can help you keep your bond secure—and can help you ensure that daycare will play a positive role in your child's life. If you feel that you and your baby are securely attached, that you are in comfortable harmony with each other, then you and your baby are ready for daycare.

You and Your Daycare Provider

Most people who choose child care as a career do so for a combination of reasons. Someone may open a family daycare business so she can stay home with her children while earning income. A woman may choose work in a daycare center because she finds nothing so fascinating as the developing minds of young children. Those that stay with their field all have in common a genuine love of children, and a rare ability to love other people's children. Professional child care offers too few monetary or social rewards and is much too challenging both mentally and physically for anyone who does not understand and adore children. Enter your search with this thought in mind, rather than with the suspicion and condescension too prevalent toward child-care providers. Sometimes when we feel new to a situation and unsure of ourselves, we find it difficult to trust others. Take care not to cast apprehensions you may have about this new stage in your life on every potential provider you meet.

> 66I need to trust my husband, my daycare provider, my parents. I even have to trust my dog to be gentle, for crying out loud. But I can't trust anyone else until I trust myself, which I don't. Of course I trust my husband and my family and the babysitter for all sorts of things, but when I'm not even sure what I expect of myself in caring for my daughter, it's hard to know what to expect of others. 99
>
> —A MOTHER IN AN ONLINE FORUM

Review your attitudes: Where do you place paid child care on your personal status ladder? Do you consider a babysitter a valued partner, or do you put her in a class with a housekeeper? Do you prefer to specify all the details of your child's care, or are you willing to let your chosen caregiver employ her experience, wisdom, and understanding of your child? The answers you arrive at will help you decide what kind of child care will work best for you and your family.

Practical considerations will affect your choice of provider. Travel time and difficulty between home, daycare, and work must be considered. Would traffic along the route be a daily aggravation? How quickly could you get to your baby in an emergency? Many mothers look for daycare near their workplaces so they can drop by in the middle of the day to nurse their babies.

You also will need to consider whether you would like to have your baby cared for in your own home, in a family daycare home, or at a daycare center. Researchers have identified three indicators of quality in any type of daycare: the number of children in a group, the amount of time they spend with the same adult, and the investment that the caregiver has made in understanding child development. Evaluate each daycare arrangement according to these basic criteria before examining the details. Also, at every daycare home or center you visit, ask whether parents are allowed to drop in unannounced. If unexpected visits are not welcomed, cross the provider off your list.

FOUR BASIC QUESTIONS FOR DAYCARE PROVIDERS

◆ How many children are in a group, and how many adults care for them? An adult should care for no more than four infants. The smaller the group, the better.

◆ How much time do the children spend with a particular adult? Staff turnover is hard on children. Ask how long caregivers have been there, and how often new staff are added.

◆ What investment has the caregiver made in understanding child development? Does the caregiver belong to an association of early-childhood educators or another professional group? Has the daycare been accredited by the National Association for the Education of Young Children or the National Association for Family Child Care? Those that are accredited have met voluntary standards for child care that are higher than most state licensing requirements.

◆ Are parents allowed to drop in unannounced?

In-Home Care

Hiring a nanny to provide care at home is the first choice of many parents. It is comforting to know that your baby is being cared for in your own home by someone undistracted by other children. It is wonderfully convenient to have someone arrive in the morning ready to take over when you need to leave for work, even if the baby isn't awake or dressed for the day yet. You don't have to pack a bag of diapers and bottles, bundle the baby up, and deliver her somewhere on the way to work. In addition, this arrangement enables you to oversee every detail of your baby's day more easily. You can decide when your baby should be taken for a walk, when she should be encouraged to take a nap and to have a bottle. You will know exactly what your baby does each day. Another advantage of having your baby cared for in your home is that she won't be exposed to other children's germs and is therefore likely to get sick less often than children in group care. Most important, when she does get sick she can stay home with a familiar caregiver without your having to stay home, too. In-home care may be a particularly good choice if your baby is just six to eight weeks old when you must go back to work. In this case, you may want to find a babysitter who can come to your home for the first few months, until your baby is older and you feel ready to investigate other possibilities. Although in-home care seems ideal, in reality it can be problematic. It is extremely expensive. Not only must you pay a full salary, but you must also pay Social Security, Medicare, and federal unemployment taxes for your nanny. Your car insurance payments may increase, if she will be using your family car. If your nanny requests it, you must withhold federal income tax from her paycheck and file her W-4 forms quarterly. You may need to increase your homeowner's insurance or buy a separate workers' compensation policy in case your babysitter is hurt on the job. Will your nanny pay for her own health insurance, ask you to pay for it, or go without? How much, if any, paid vacation time will you offer? Will her sick days be paid? You must decide all these things, and keep the necessary records.

Most problems with in-home care, however, have to do with the nanny's enjoyment of the job and her relationship with her employers. Unless the nanny is a recluse, she may feel too isolated in this sort of job. If she knows other nannies or mothers in the neighborhood, she can meet them at playgrounds and in backyards to relieve some of the loneliness. But even nannies who manage to socialize this way often move on to other jobs within the first year. Often, they quit because of an unhappy relationship with the parents.

The fact is that someone who excels at child care is likely to value relationships so much that she considers them to *be* her work. Lynn Manfredi/Petitt, a family daycare provider, writes in the journal *Young Children,* "The repetitiveness of chores, delayed gratification of accomplishments, and lack of money seem less important to those who place a priority on relationships. . . . The promise and adventure of authentic, long-term relationships encourage many people to consider spending their days with children for a living," and compensate those who stay in the business. Unfortunately, the providers' special abilities are "virtually invisible; therefore, many people (including caregivers themselves) have difficulty seeing beyond the common assumption that child-care providers are paid for doing the chores involved." Many people, Manfredi/Petitt continues, "believe that *just about anyone can do the job* of caring for other people's children. Clearly a new awareness is in order: Professional caregiving is a specialized skill based on the ability to love beyond genetic bonds." If you want your caregiver to stay and to be happy in her job, be aware that the quality of your relationship with her is an essential part of her compensation package.

If you have space for someone to live in your home, consider an au pair. Young women, and sometimes men, are recruited by several established U.S. agencies to live with American families for a year (yes, you would need to welcome a new, different au pair at the end of the year). Most often from Europe, au pairs come from the Middle East, South Africa, and other parts of the United States as well. Screened and trained before their arrival, au pairs want to learn English, take classes at a local college, and enjoy family life in another culture. For this opportunity (and for approximately one thousand dollars per month, plus air fare, room and board, and agency fees), au pairs can provide as much as 45 hours of child care in your home each week. You may instead find your own au pair through family or friends, but you won't have an agency's guarantee that, if things don't work out for one reason or another, a different au pair will show up within 30 days.

Run under the auspices of the U.S. State Department, the Au Pair Program enables citizens of other countries between 18 and 26 years of age to live with host families in exchange for providing limited child-care services for up to 12 months. An au pair's working hours are limited to 10 hours per day and 45 hours per week. An au pair cannot be placed with a family having an infant less than three months old unless a parent or other responsible adult stays home. Au pairs placed in homes with children under two years of age must have at least 200 hours of experience caring for infants.

If you want to try an au pair, remember that this person caring for your child will not be a household employee but a temporary member of your family. Remember, too, that most au pairs are in their late teens or early twenties, still adolescents in many ways. Although generally well trained in child care, they may need someone to watch over them. Be prepared to help heal homesickness or a broken heart. Don't be surprised at finding yourself parenting a teenager on occasion, including setting limits on use of the car and weekend activities. Remember, too, that taking care of a young baby all day is hard work, especially if the caretaker is relatively young herself. Be sure that your au pair gets the rest and support she needs, and that the job does not overwhelm her.

Despite the occasional au pair disaster story, the arrangement is often a delight for everyone involved. A family now hosting their fifth au pair declares, "Choosing the au pair route was one of the best things we ever did. Thanks to that choice, we now have a bilingual (in German and English) four-year-old who can find more countries on a globe than most adults, several extended families in Europe, and a wonderful, lively house."

> "Interview an au pair by phone extensively, in her own language if possible. Most importantly, know that an au pair gives you what you give her. If you treat her as a babysitter, that is what you will get. If you treat her as a member of the family, you will be rewarded with a rich experience, a loving caregiver, and a lifetime friend."
>
> —PARENT HOST OF AN AU PAIR

Another sensible variant on in-home care is shared care. In this arrangement, two or more families who live near one another hire someone to take care of their children together. In this way the caregiver makes more money than she would with one child, and the parents pay less than they would for one-on-one care. This arrangement is wonderful for the children, who even as babies enjoy having a buddy to play with every day. The arrangement can also be a lot more fun for the caregiver. Some families alternate the house in which the children and the caregiver stay, by the week or by the month; some use one house exclusively. The host family may pay slightly less than its partner family. In some arrangements, the caregivers are the parents, who tend to all the babies on a round-robin schedule.

Either way, sharing baby care with another family means building and tending twice as many long-term relationships: Getting along well with the other child's parents is as essential as having a good relationship with the caregiver. The parents need to agree about how they would like the caregiver to handle matters such as naps, meals, and outings. If you would like your baby to have the freedom to explore the house when he begins to crawl, and the other family would like their baby to spend his day securely limited to one childproof room, you may run into difficulties.

If you decide that in-home care is the right choice for you, search for the right person along as many avenues as possible. Place a classified ad in your local paper (review the other ads first to inform yourself about going rates and other standards for your area). Write your ad to appeal to the person you have in mind—warm, well-organized, honest. Tell everyone you know that you are looking for a good babysitter; if you find a person recommended by someone you trust, you've struck gold. Put notices up in local colleges and senior centers; lonely retirees can make wonderful substitute grandmothers. If you can afford the fees, consider hiring a nanny through a reputable professional agency.

When you find a prospective caregiver, find out the basics. What is her previous child-care experience? Does she have references? Does she have a valid driver's license? Is she willing to take a tuberculosis test, or has she had one recently? Does she know infant CPR (or is she willing to take a class in it at your expense)? Then ask the essential questions, phrasing them in ways that will not put her on the defensive:

◆ Why is she interested in this job?

◆ Does she enjoy child care, or does she perceive it as a job to do until something better comes along?

◆ Would she be willing to carry your baby in a baby pack or sling, even for much of the day, if the baby is happier that way?

◆ How does she feel about crying babies? Should they be picked up right away or left to cry?

◆ How does she feel about breastfeeding, and how does she react to the thought of handling breast milk?

Throughout your interview, keep in mind the most important quality a caregiver should have—the ability to build a loving relationship with your child—and consider all other factors afterward. Look for someone who values relationships and is gifted at forming them. If you and your sitter form a successful match, not only will you avoid having to launch another search in a short while, but, most importantly, your baby will benefit from having a consistent, loving substitute caregiver.

Relatives

Substitute care provided by a relative, usually the baby's grandmother or an aunt, can be heaven or a disaster. Some grandparents feel exploited in this role; others wouldn't want their grandchildren to be cared for by anyone else. In traditional societies, of course, caring for children and teaching them cultural lore are primary responsibilities of the elderly. When parents and their parents both favor this form of substitute care, it can serve as the basis of marvelously strong intergenerational ties.

Before accepting your relative's offer to provide daycare, consider how much she respects your new status as a parent and, especially, your decision to breastfeed. While you are at work, will your relative care for your baby as you do, or are her style and philosophy at odds with your own? Will she pick up your baby when he cries? Will she be able to carry your baby in a frontpack or sling? Will she be comfortable handling your stored breast milk and feeding it to your baby? Does she know about breastfeeding and its benefits, or is she willing to learn? Does she support your decision to work? You know this person well, which is a tremendous advantage; use that knowledge as you consider the likely consequences of sharing baby care with her.

If you are considering an arrangement with a relative, don't assume she wouldn't like to be paid. Paying for a job well done is a sign of respect, and respect is the key to making this arrangement work.

Family Daycare

Family daycare can be a wonderful option, too. In most states, a licensed family daycare provider can care for as many as six or, if she has an assistant, ten children, with a maximum of four infants, in her own home. The group is usually of mixed ages, typically between a few months and three or four years. This grouping of mixed-age children under the consistent care of one or two adults is much like the way most children have been cared for throughout human history.

Many parents choose family daycare primarily because it offers a home environment. The provider's family members may come and go throughout the day. The postman arrives, and the telephone rings. Lunch is in the kitchen, and naps are on beds. Ideally, the provider's home becomes a second home for your child, just as familiar and warm and safe as your own.

You can find family daycare homes in your area by calling or e-mailing a child-care resource or referral organization. (See Resources, pages 218–19, for Web addresses for these national organizations.) You can also scan bulletin boards in libraries, schools, churches, and child-oriented businesses; read the newspaper's classified section; and ask parents of slightly older children for their recommendations. If your state maintains a registry of licensed daycare providers, obtain a list of all those in your zip code. If you would like to nurse your baby during the workday, ask for a list of providers in the zip code of your workplace as well.

When you interview a prospective daycare provider, try to discern her attitudes about her work, about the children in her care, and about the parents of those children:

- How many years has she been providing family daycare?
- Does she take her work seriously, or is it simply a way for her to supplement her family's income without having to leave the house?

◆ How much does she know–through education, experience, or intuition–about child development?

◆ Does the provider belong to any professional groups, receive newsletters, or take classes in child development? Is she a member of the National Association for Family Child Care?

◆ Is she licensed by the state? (Remember, though, that licensing does not guarantee excellent care. Accreditation by the National Association for the Education of Young Children or other professional group is a more reliable measure of quality.)

◆ Does the provider's daily schedule include time outdoors, a midmorning snack, planned activities, nap time, and no TV?

◆ Does the daycare hold family gatherings and reach out to become your social center as well as your substitute care? Will it be possible to view this place, in time, as an extension of you and your baby's home and family?

When you visit a prospective family daycare home, observe carefully:

◆ Is it clean and hazard-free?

◆ Does it have a safe outdoor play area, away from streets?

◆ Where do the children eat and nap?

Observe the provider as she interacts with the children in her care:

◆ How does she handle a two-year-old who is having a rough day?

◆ How does she care for a baby at the same time?

◆ Are the children engaged and happy in their activities?

◆ Are they comfortable and familiar with the provider?

◆ Is she positive and warm with them?

◆ While you and she talk, does she break off the conversation frequently to attend to their needs?

If the answer to the last question is yes, good. This provider has her priorities straight.

As you chat, consider whether you can form a mutually supportive relationship with this provider. Can you learn from her years of experience with children? Will she respect your point of view? Will she be a positive influence in your child's life? Call the parents with whom the provider now works and ask them to talk about their best and worst experiences with the daycare home. Observe, if you can, pick-up time at the daycare. How do the parents and the provider greet each other? Does she share information about their children's day with them? Do they seem comfortable together?

If you like what you see, talk in depth with the provider about how you feel your baby should be cared for. Tell her you breastfeed, but let her respond before you go further. If she is informed about breast-feeding and supportive, wonderful. If she did not nurse her own children and knows little about breastfeeding, consider whether you'll be able to enlist her support. She must be willing to keep your pumped milk in her freezer and to thaw it for your baby's meals. You must be comfortable nursing your baby in her home. If she would rather not see a mother nurse in her living room, you may need to look else-where.

But if you sense that the provider is not disapproving of breast-feeding but simply uninformed on the subject, you might offer her something to read on the importance of breastfeeding and the bene-fits of breast milk. Nurse discreetly in front of her so she becomes more comfortable with breastfeeding. One mother describes the process of converting her child's caregiver: "I'm the only nursing mother in the five families she works with, and I've nursed longer than any other mother she has known. She knows very little about nursing and expressed breast milk, but I've been slowly making com-ments and educating her about the differences. It's obvious to me that she probably prefers the ease (for her) of formula, but she is becoming more and more supportive as time goes on."

Once you know you have your provider's support for breastfeeding in general, talk about the details of feeding your baby. Explain that you'd like the bottle feeding of your pumped milk to mimic breastfeeding as much as possible. You would like your baby to be fed in the provider's arms, for example, rather than in a seat with a propped bottle. You would like her fed when she seems hungry rather than on a rigid schedule. Tell the provider, though, that you would prefer she not give the baby a bottle just before you arrive to pick her up, since you'll want her to be eager to nurse (although she probably will be no matter what). Depending on the proximity of the daycare home to your workplace, you may wish to nurse your baby during your lunch hour; if so, ask how the provider feels about this. Talk about solid foods, too, so she knows when and how you would like them to be introduced into your baby's diet. Later you can give the provider detailed instructions on storing, thawing, and feeding breast milk (see page 155).

If your baby is happiest being carried, find out how the provider feels about this. Is she willing to wear the baby in a sling or a baby pack? Wear the baby yourself while visiting with your provider to demonstrate how comfortable and easy it is. Point out how free your hands are, and how content your baby is.

Ask about nap times, too. If one day your baby doesn't seem to want or need her nap, or wants to be held instead of laid down, will the provider accommodate her needs?

When you're sure that you and the provider are compatible, talk with her about practical details—

◆ How and when does she want to be paid?

◆ What if you arrive a little late to pick up the baby one day?

◆ Will you pay if your child is sick and cannot come for a day or two?

◆ What if the provider gets sick? Does she still get paid?

◆ Does she collect holiday pay?

◆ Do you pay when you go on vacation? Does she get paid when she goes on vacation, and when does she go?

An established daycare provider will have ready answers for all these questions. If your chosen provider hasn't set policies, work out mutually agreeable plans ahead of time. Leaving a daycare arrangement that is falling apart because of disagreements and quickly finding a new one quickly tops the list of worst nightmares for working parents. So be fair as you work out these arrangements. Your daycare provider may want the same paid holidays most employed people receive, or she may set her rates high enough to cover her holidays. She needs vacations, paid or not, more than most people (her days are long and she lives in her workplace). If your child wakes up with chicken pox and can't go to her house, she should still be paid.

Remember that your daycare provider is offering you the most important service possible: help in raising your child. If you have chosen well, the provider will be a ready source of seasoned advice who knows your child nearly as well as you do. Daycare providers often step into the role of the experienced relatives and neighbors who once supplied the parenting wisdom new mothers needed then and still need now. Respect that the provider's work takes place in her own home, where you will always be a guest even though you are paying for her service. Ideally, a family daycare provider is treated with the same sensitivity, affection, and tolerance as the baby's grandparent or aunt. You'll want to let your provider know often how much you appreciate the work she does.

Daycare Centers

Daycare centers offer both the best and the worst of modern child care. They can be homey, nurturing places with staffs that understand child development and are well trained in caring for children with varying needs. Or they can be impersonal, rigidly organized institutions. You'll know the difference when you see it. The great advantage of daycare centers is their reliability. You can count on a daycare center to be available every day that you must work.

The great disadvantage of using a daycare center is your child's chance of contracting infections there. A study published in 2005 showed that children under two years old in large daycare centers are 36 times more likely than children who stay at home to contract pneumococcal infections (a leading cause of earaches), pneumonia, and meningitis. The risk for children in family daycare of catching the same infections is just 4.4 times greater than for those who are cared for in their homes, the researchers found. Dr. Ben Schwartz, an epidemiologist with the Centers for Disease Control and Prevention, recommends that parents who rely on daycare centers counteract this increased chance of infection by keeping their children away from cigarette smoke, by maintaining good hygiene, and by breastfeeding.

Infant care in a center must be scrutinized with particular care. Sit in a corner of the room for a good half hour or more, and watch how the babies are handled:

- What is the ratio of adults to babies? It should be no more than one to four, with a maximum of eight to ten babies in each group.

- Are the adults holding, rocking, and playing with the babies? Or are the babies tucked into swings and walkers and playpens except when they need to be fed or diapered?

- How consistent is the care? Does each staff member take primary responsibility for certain babies? Will there be one person whom your baby will recognize as his caregiver when you drop him off in the morning?

Ask the same questions of the staff at a center that you would of a family daycare provider. You should be able to find support for breastfeeding at a daycare center. You should be able to drop in at any time to nurse your baby, if you wish. And you should be able to develop close, mutually supportive relationships with the staff members who will be caring for your baby while you work.

Most centers group children by age, combining the two- and three-year-olds in one room and the four- and five-year-olds in another room. Check out these rooms, too, if possible. If you're very lucky, your first daycare arrangement will be your last. If you like this place, you will probably want your child to stay in it at least until preschool and perhaps until kindergarten (some large centers even offer a kindergarten year). What are the older children doing? Are they happily engaged in a variety of projects and imaginative play? Do the teachers sit on the floor to play with the children, and kneel or squat so they can talk with the children face to face? If artwork, posters, and decorations are at your eye level rather than the children's, the center may be more concerned with impressing visiting parents than with enriching the children's days.

Some centers are experimenting with "family groupings," mixing two- to five-year-olds in small groups with one teacher in charge. As in a family daycare home, a neighborhood full of children, or a village, the younger children learn from the older ones, and the older ones enjoy teaching the little ones, learning nurturing skills as they do so. If you find a center with such groupings, observe for a while to see how you like them.

Corporate on-site daycare centers are often touted as the perfect solution to the work-and-family dilemma. American businesses are certainly taking a step in the right direction when they assume a share of the responsibility for helping parents combine work and child raising. Beware, however, of the company-run daycare center that is the pet project of the public-relations department rather than the human-resources department. A mother who works for one large corporation shares her experience: "My company provides on-site daycare—if you can ever get in. The waiting list is huge. I put my name on when I was three months pregnant, and my daughter is now four years old. We never got in. This is especially frustrating since the company makes a big deal in the press about its working mother-friendly policy." If you do get your child into an on-site daycare center, there will be the potential problem of having to change centers if you decide to change jobs.

Backup Plans

Whatever child-care arrangement you decide upon, know that the day will come when you need substitute care for your substitute care. Your in-home babysitter gets the flu. Your family daycare provider's mother is having surgery in another state. Your daycare center is closing for three weeks in the summer. Your baby wakes up with a fever and must stay home for the day. What you do in these situations depends very much on your job. Having the flexibility to take the day off or to work at home will make your life infinitely easier. But having backup arrangements also will ease your mind. Do your baby's grandparents live near by? Are they willing to step in in a pinch? How cozy are you with the other parents on your street? Is there an at-home mother who might be willing to be there for you *once in a while* if she knows you'll be there for her on a Saturday night? Bringing your baby to work with you is another possibility not to be casually dismissed. The ins and outs of managing this are discussed in Chapter 7.

Preparing Your Home and Family

About two weeks before your first day back at work, you may wish to take a few other steps to ensure that the transition causes you as little stress as possible. Expect the first weeks back at work to have much in common with the first weeks of motherhood. Consider this a second postpartum period, during which you will need the same care and concern as when your baby was born. Small events will loom large, as they did in that first week. Fatigue will be a familiar companion as you learn to manage both work and mothering. For now, prepare your home much as you may have done in the weeks before your baby was born. Cook several main dishes, and freeze them. Stock up on nutritious foods that can be prepared quickly. Consider asking a friend or relative to help out. If there's a grocery delivery service in your area, this may be the time to give it a try. Often these services allow you to order your groceries online and have them delivered the same day for a nominal fee. A woman whose mother came to help when her baby was born asked her mother-in-law to come for her first week back at work. Just as you did after giving birth, you will need both emotional support and physical assistance with household and child-care chores, and as much rest as possible.

Your mate can make all the difference during this transition period. If he truly bears at least 50 percent of the household duties, you are already a long way toward meeting the challenge of working and mothering. Unfortunately, many husbands support their wives' return to work and say they'll help out, but don't really comprehend what needs to be done. While women tend to accept this inequity to keep the peace, they also are more likely to suffer with chronic exhaustion, low sex drive, and frequent illness.

Talk with your spouse as frankly as you can about how the two of you will manage household tasks. Be clear about the difference between helping out and taking full responsibility. Does cooking dinner mean just that, or does it include the planning, shopping, and cleanup? Does getting the dry cleaning done mean simply dropping the clothes off at the cleaners on the way to work, or does it mean collecting the clothes, bringing them in with instructions for special treatment, keeping track of the receipt, and picking them up on time—all without being reminded? In many marriages in which the husband comfortably takes credit for half the domestic tasks, neither he nor his wife acknowledges the weight of the details surrounding each of the wife's tasks. Going back to work does not mean that everything is back to normal and that you are ready to do everything you did before. In your first six months back at work, as in your first days at home with your baby, you will need to focus on caring for yourself and your baby during all your off hours. Your mate can make this possible.

Preparing Your Workplace

The Economist reported in 2005 that women account for almost half the work force in companies in industrialized nations. In the executive suites, however, there are still ten men for every woman. Why the difference? There may still be lingering doubts that a woman can do the job, whatever the job may be, but the primary reason for the lack of women at the top is that women bear children. They take time off when their babies are born, or, frequently, when their children's lives become complicated by after-school activities. Families require flexibility to meet these needs, and women usually supply it. Although many women return to work after a few years, corporate culture remains intolerant of mid-career absences. One study of American managers found that women returning to work after a break of three years or more lost an average of 37 percent of their earning power.

Change is in the air, however, as an increasing number of corporations realize that keeping women on board and making it possible for them to reach the top echelons is good for the bottom line. Research has shown a strong correlation between shareholder returns and the proportion of women at the executive level. A corporate culture that understands the different pace and path of women's careers can produce more profits than one that forces all employees into the same mold. Investment in flexibility has become a new principle of good business.

These corporations have observed that women make special contributions. Women tend to be skilled communicators and devoted team builders. Especially if they are mothers, women tend to see the long view, and keep issues in perspective. They work hard when time is short, and waste little time at the water cooler. Because they have lives outside of work, they understand the real needs and desires of the customers the corporation seeks to serve.

Firms that understand the value of women in their work force are on the forefront of meeting the challenges of combining work and mothering, especially the challenge of returning to work after a baby is born. "Phase-back" policies, which allow new mothers to gradually resume a full work schedule, flexible hours for all parents and for employees with elders to care for, and telecommuting have all made it possible for companies to keep valued employees. Parents who don't stay long into the evening or hop on a plane at a moment's notice are not necessarily penalized in pay, advancement, or respect.

When you return to your workplace, keep these observations in mind. Sometimes our own fears become reality when we too easily accept the misperceptions of others. Don't allow a colleague or manager to convince you that your new role as a mother should reduce your status or effectiveness in the workplace.

First Days Back: Finding Pumping Space

If you don't have access to a private office and aren't sure where else you can pump, stop by your workplace "just to say hello," and scout out a good pumping place before your maternity leave ends. If there is no designated "lactation room" for nursing mothers, schedule a talk with your human resources department. Meeting this essential need of their employees is part of their job, and they need to locate a clean and private place for you to pump your milk. That place may be a dedicated room, a private office, or a women's locker room. Conference rooms, storage rooms, and nurse's offices have all been used by nursing moms. Bathrooms should not be even a last resort. Don't let someone bully you into using a toilet stall because he or she equates breast milk with other bodily fluids. You are preparing a meal for your baby, and you deserve an appropriate place in which to do so. Some mothers without other options have found that the best place for pumping is one's own car in the parking lot. With a sun-shade across the front and a towel or two draped across the windows, your car can be private and, because it is your own place, relaxing.

If no suitable pumping place is available, you may want to persuade your company to create one. Consider how you will make your proposal. Depending on the culture of your company, you may need to present your proposal in a way that highlights the benefits to the company of supporting nursing mothers. In any case, you'll want to take care to avoid setting off alarm bells about your commitment to your job without giving into pressures to hide your motherhood. How you'll make your request may depend on your own sense of your rights and value as an employee and parent.

Your Legal Rights

Inform your request for a pumping space with knowledge of your legal rights, as well. "Breastfeeding legislation" is on the rise, with federal and state laws being passed and proposed. The laws tend to address one of three issues: the right of mothers to nurse their babies in public, excusing nursing mothers from jury service, and the right of employed mothers to nurse or express their milk during working hours.

With the exception of federal legislation introduced by U.S. Representative Carolyn Maloney of New York, these are state laws, and they vary considerably. Depending on where you live, you have may explicit, implied, or no legal protection at all. New York was the first state to enact comprehensive breastfeeding legislation, which it did in 1984. This legislation excepted breastfeeding in public from the criminal statutes for indecent exposure and disorderly conduct. Following suit in 1993, Florida enacted a law that identified breastfeeding as an important and basic act of nature that should be encouraged in the interests of maternal and child health. The law provided that a woman had a right to breastfeed in any place where she had a right to be. Thirty-three other states modeled laws after these and, at this writing, several more have pending bills dealing with the protection of breastfeeding.

Less common are laws that specifically protect the rights of working women to nurse or express their milk at their place of work. Hawaii prohibits employers from discriminating against a mother who breastfeeds or expresses milk at work. Just six states, Connecticut, California, Georgia, Illinois, Minnesota, and Tennessee, require that employers provide break time and private accommodations for employees to express breast milk for their babies, or "make a reasonable effort to do so." At this writing, only California, Georgia, and Tennessee specify that the location cannot be a toilet stall. California alone requires that all state employees be allowed to breastfeed or express milk during working hours. Texas has a law that "encourages" employers to allow working women to express their breast milk during working hours, by promising cooperative employers the official designation of "mother friendly." Nationally, the right to breastfeed is under discussion. The Right to Breastfeed Act, introduced by Rep. Maloney, ensures a woman's right to nurse her child anywhere on federal property where she and her child are authorized to be. A clarification to the Pregnancy Discrimination Act of 1999 would protect breastfeeding under civil rights law, by stating that women cannot be fired or discriminated against in the workplace for expressing their breast milk or breastfeeding during a break. At this writing, this bill remains under consideration by a congressional committee. Rep. Maloney has also introduced acts that would provide tax incentives for businesses that establish private lactation areas in the workplace, establish a performance standard for breast pumps, and make breastfeeding equipment tax-deductible (at this writing, these acts are in committee). The U.S. Senate is considering the Help America Act to promote overall public health; it includes a section requiring employers to provide "lactation periods and facilities" for employees who are breastfeeding.

The Profit Motive

If you live in one of the few states with an enacted law requiring your employer to provide private pumping space for nursing employees, your task is relatively straightforward. You must make your employer, or your human resources department, aware of the necessity of complying with the law. If your state has no law to protect breast-feeding workers, you may need to pull together a list of reasons that supporting the nursing mothers on the staff makes good business sense. Besides explaining the overall value of accommodating the needs of women in the company work force, highlight the financial benefits of meeting the needs of nursing mothers:

◆ Reduced absenteeism. Breastfeeding mothers lose less time from the workplace because breastfed babies tend to stay healthier than their formula-fed counterparts.

◆ Lower turnover. Supporting employees' need to pump milk for 6 to 12 months creates enduring employee loyalty at low cost.

◆ Potential savings in health-care expenditures.

◆ Tax benefits. With passage of certain federal bills now under consideration, employers will receive incentives for establishing lactation facilities on their premises.

Does your employer use a work-life consulting agency? Many medium to large companies contract much of their human-resources work out to this growing industry, to provide their employees with assistance in staying healthy, finding child and elder care, and other personal and family needs. Increasingly, these firms also provide lactation support services. LifeCare: Life Event Management Services, for example, offers a program called "Mothers at Work" that provides pregnant and breastfeeding employees with round-the-clock counseling by lactation consultants, educational materials, breast pumps, and other equipment. These services may already be on your roster of benefits. If not, your company may be persuaded to consider them, with or without the help of a work-life agency.

What do you need specifically to express your milk at work?

- ◆ 15- to 30-minute breaks two to three times a day, or once every three hours. If you will nurse your baby at a nearby daycare home or center rather than expressing your milk, you will need 30 minutes twice a day. (Depending on your state and the kind of work you do, all employees already may be allowed 15-minute breaks every two hours. If so, you may be able to arrange an alternative schedule of fewer but slightly longer breaks.)

- ◆ A clean, private place with a locking door that is not a toilet stall or adjacent to one.

- ◆ A comfortable chair and a small table for a breast pump.

- ◆ An electrical outlet.

- ◆ A sink to wash hands and rinse equipment.

- ◆ A refrigerator for milk storage.

- ◆ A nonharassment policy for breastfeeding mothers.

These requirements may last from three months to a year.

Keep in mind that the accommodations for which you're asking will make a great deal of difference to you and your baby and little difference, most likely, to your employer.

If there is more than one nursing mother at work, you will gain ground by joining forces in your proposal. Include an outline of how employees will coordinate use of the lactation space. Will you set up a schedule for use among yourselves? Will you use a whiteboard on the outside of the door to note who is in the room and how long she expects to be there? Who will keep the space clean and organized? Fill in all the details so that your employer can see how smoothly things will run.

Extending Your Maternity Leave

According to the Pregnancy Discrimination Act and the Family Medical Leave Act, you have a right to six weeks of maternity leave with disability pay (less than full pay) plus six more weeks without pay—if your employer has 50 or more employees, and if you have worked for that employer at least 25 hours per week for the year preceding your leave. If your employer offers only these minimum maternity benefits (or if you're ineligible even for these), and you want to extend your leave to three or four months, you have some negotiating to do. Your success will depend on how valuable you are to your employer and how flexible company policies are. Consider enlisting your doctor's support to drive home the importance of establishing a close attachment to your baby through full-time breastfeeding before returning to work. Come armed with the names of comparable companies that allow longer leaves; most profitable companies do.

Alternative Work Arrangements

No matter how long your maternity leave, when it's over you may not feel ready to put your baby in daycare from dawn to dusk five days a week. Consider whether one of these innovative arrangements might be the solution:

First, you might ask your employer for a flexible schedule. **Flextime** has become a standard at many companies, thanks to the requests of desperate and determined parents and employees with elderly parents of their own. In 2005, according to one survey, 67 percent of working parents report they have some flexibility on the job. Usually, employees can start and finish work when they prefer, as long as they are on the job during core working hours, such as 10:00 A.M. to 3:00 P.M. If both parents are lucky enough to work on flextime schedules, one can leave for work early and come home early, while the other leaves later and comes home later, so that the baby need spend only four or five hours in daycare.

Stanley Greenspan, M.D., a physician and an expert in infant and child development, suggests yet another flexible arrangement. In his book *The Four-Thirds Solution: Solving the Childcare Crisis in America Today*, he encourages parents to rearrange their work schedules to allow more time at home. The core of his idea is that each parent work two-thirds time (about 27 hours a week) on different days of the week, or overlapping by one day. With this schedule, each parent is home one-third of the workweek, and substitute child care is minimized or nonexistent. Blend a home office into the mix and the flexibility to work when the baby is sleeping, and the scenario seems even more productive and appealing. Less pie-in-the-sky than it might have been just a few years ago, Greenspan's idea has numerous practical variations, and families of all sorts are putting them into action.

Compressed workweeks for full-time employees are also gaining in popularity; you might work four 10-hour days followed by three days off, or three 12-hour days followed by four days off. Airline flight attendants and pilots, many with babies at home, follow schedules like these. Such a schedule could be stressful, though. Your workdays would be long and tiring, and your days off might also have a wearying intensity if you are trying to make up for lost time. You would need to pump at least three and probably four times each workday. Compressed workweeks divide a person's life cleanly in two, with work and home hardly mixing at all. Many people feel comfortable with this and prefer it to the usual schedule, but consider carefully how you would find the weekly transitions before suggesting a compressed workweek to your employer.

Telecommuting may be a nearly ideal solution for combining work and mothering. Thanks to the Internet and other wonders of our age, you can be in contact with your coworkers while at home almost as easily as if you were at work. One woman describes her situation: "My boss was wonderful to let me work at home for the last two months of a difficult pregnancy. I still work at home now several times a week, but in order to manage it with my boss, I provide her with a weekly report of what I've accomplished. I also check voice mail and e-mail messages several times a day. We periodically go over goals and achievement to make sure it works well. I still have to put my kids in daycare when I'm home, but the benefit is that I can pick them up when I'm done with my work—usually around 2:30—rather than at the end of the workday and a long commute."

Telecommuting arrangements can be a boon to business as well. At one Aetna Health Plans division, telecommuting has increased the productivity of claims processors by 29 percent. Workers are also making fewer errors, and the company is saving thousands on office space.

Although working at home would allow you more time with your baby, you might miss the casual interaction with your colleagues—and they might eventually decide that they really do need you in person. Another woman recalls, "I worked out of my home for six months after my son was born, via computer, fax, and phone. When I suggested extending the arrangement, my company said they preferred to see my face full time. It comes down to their being able to pop their heads into my office with a simple question." Telecommuting may work well enough, however, until your baby is older and you feel more comfortable being separated.

Part-time work may be a solution for you, if you can afford it. Although your income would decrease, so would your daycare expenses. Is there a part of your job that you do especially well and for which your employer most values you? Write a proposal redesigning your job into a part-time position dedicated to that function, with prorated pay and benefits. Be sure to negotiate an hourly rate, so that if you put in extra hours you'll get paid for them. You might propose that you work an average of 20 hours a week, with an annual maximum of 1,000 hours, so that your schedule can fluctuate to meet the needs of your workplace and your family.

If your employer agrees to a part-time schedule, be prepared for changes in the way your colleagues and managers perceive you. You may find that you are not taken as seriously as you were before, or that you've lost some of the perks that went with your previous position, such as the parking place or a company cell phone. You may find you can't advance as a part-timer. One manager for a large insurance company writes, "In my experience, part-time employees are often treated like second-class citizens. The men in management tend to think their heart is no longer in their career. I'm treated as if I no longer want to be in the fast track or considered for promotion. I am someone who moved up rapidly, but the corporate culture still makes me feel this way."

Sitting on a plateau for a few years, however, won't necessarily keep you from eventually reaching career heights. A government lawyer has no regrets about her choice to work part time while her children were babies: "When my children were five and three, I returned to work full time and have since been promoted twice. My children have always been well cared for, and I have a husband who believes that he is as responsible for their care as I am. I am very happy with the choices I made and continue to make. Promotion may take longer, and people in the workplace need to be convinced that you really care, but it is possible." If there is ever a time in your life when you might want to ease your career's trajectory a bit while still keeping your foot in the door, now is probably it.

Job sharing is a part-time work arrangement that often makes sense for both employer and employee. In this arrangement, two employees manage the responsibilities of one position. Often one person works Monday through Wednesday and the other Wednesday through Friday; they catch up with each other on the overlapping day. The employer benefits from having two energetic employees, and all the experience and resources they both bring to the job, for the price of one overextended employee. The employees divide the benefits and the salary in a way that works for them and their firm. Ideally, the job-sharing partners are flexible enough to step in for each other when one misses work because of a sick child or vacation.

To pursue any of these arrangements, your first step is to write a confident, convincing proposal for your employer. Describe the arrangement you desire, its benefits to your employer, and how you would handle situations that might arise.

Staying Home Instead

What if you are about to go back to work but every cell in your body is screaming that this is not what you want to do? And yet the alternative, quitting and staying at home full time, just doesn't seem workable? There's the loss of income, for starters. Long gone are the days when a working mother's income was for the "extras," the family's fun money for vacations and a second car. Your income is more likely to pay the mortgage or the rent, and to cover groceries, college savings, and other necessities. You may also be uncomfortable with the idea of walking away from your career and your life outside the home. Who will you be without your professional identity? Will your mind turn to mush? Will you go stir-crazy? What will you do when your children are no longer small?

The first step to finding the answers is to develop an appreciation for the creative pleasures and intellectual demands of mothering. Doing so will help give you the flexibility to broaden your choices between "working" and "not working." Mothers who have made the decision to stay home after years of working in jobs they enjoyed say that many of the assumptions made about staying at home just aren't true. Listen to one: "As someone who had always worked, I struggled with the decision of whether to quit. I eased out of it. At first, I gave up my management position for a part-time position with the same company. (In other words, they thought a part-timer couldn't handle that much responsibility.) But as my second child came along and my first went into kindergarten, I knew I had to try the stay-at-home thing. It has been wonderful, and it's true, even if the kids are playing while you're doing chores, they are just enjoying being in their own environment with their own stuff and you in the background. It is a major security thing for them. At least that's how I've found it. No regrets so far. I also worried that I would be bored, bored, bored, but, just like the kids, I'm not. Quite the opposite. One thing to remember is, if you quit, it's not permanent, you can always go back. Give yourself the opportunity to make an informed decision."

Life is long, and childhood is brief. If you step out of your career path for a few years, you can step back into it later and perhaps follow new directions that you hadn't considered before. That's not to say that the progress of your career won't be altered by leaving it for a few years. Your field will evolve, and the colleagues you have left behind will advance during your absence. But in a decade or so, they may be burned out and thinking about a change, while you will be hitting your prime with a maturity earned through motherhood. To keep from feeling adrift, you might design a 10-year plan. What would you like to be doing in 10 years, when your child is on the verge of adolescence? How can you prepare for that goal, year by year, as he grows?

And what about the financial issues? There may be more leeway here than you imagine. First of all, you might consider turning some of your specialized skills into a freelance or consulting business. As corporations "downsize," they increasingly rely on outsiders to provide services formerly done by staff members. Editors, writers, public-relations specialists, designers, accountants, and computer experts are just a few of the professionals who have found a demand for their independent services. Your own company may jump at the chance to employ your expertise without having to pay the overhead costs of office space, insurance, and other benefits. You will lose those benefits, of course, but if you have a partner whose benefits include health insurance, perhaps for a few years you can manage. (Health insurance can also be obtained through membership in professional associations.) Flexibility and time at home with your child is your compensation package now.

Equate cutting back expenses with earning income; every dollar you save is indeed a dollar earned. Begin with your current salary. Now add up all the costs of working, including daycare, clothes, commuting costs, and taxes, and subtract them. Take the sum that is left, and subtract the cost of everything you now spend money on that you can possibly do without. (Do take into account the expected and unexpected costs of having a child, from life insurance to emergency-room visits.) What remains? Is it an amount that you can earn in various ways without relying on a full-time job? Is it an amount you and your family can manage without for a few years? Numerous books are full of clever ideas for reducing expenses. Take a look at *Staying Home Instead: How to Balance Your Family Life (and Your Checkbook)*, by Christine Davidson. As one mother writes, "If you really want to stay home, find a way. I was certain we could never afford it, as my paycheck paid more than half of the mortgage, but it is amazing what you can do!"

ON YOUR OWN:
FREELANCE BUSINESSES IN DEMAND

Graphic design, podcasting, illustration, photography and videography, indexing, technical writing, journalism, editing, copyediting, proofreading, transcription, webmaster, medical transcription, legal services, public-relations consulting, grant writing, sales, tax-form preparation, accounting, financial planning, mortgage brokering, property management, architecture, interior decorating, catering, massage, pet care, cleaning, tutoring, daycare, nursery or greenhouse operation, "reassurance" services for the elderly and house-bound, postpartum care, labor support, childbirth education, managing book and software fairs at schools, educational and college admissions counseling, CPR and first-aid teaching, crafts, landscape architecture, and garden design—and more!

No one of the work options described here is right for everyone. Design your life in a way that is right for you. And remember, whatever your choice, if you're happy, your baby will be happy, too.

six

BABY'S LUNCH: EXPRESSING, STORING, AND FEEDING BREAST MILK

Why Pump?

LONG BEFORE *working mother* became a common term, women found ways to express and store breast milk when nursing their babies wasn't practical or possible. Weak or sick babies needed to be fed with a teaspoon; mothers required relief from engorgement; or they needed to be elsewhere while their babies were cared for at home. Primitive pumps have been made at least since the 1800s. Nursing mothers have hand-expressed their milk, used the most awkward of pumps, and, in recent years, sent their fresh milk home to their babies by overnight express.

No matter where they have been or what they have been doing, women have found ingenious ways to give their milk to their babies. A postal worker found a daycare provider on her route, so that she could stop in and nurse her baby while delivering the mail. A traveling sales rep plugged an electric pump into the cigarette lighter in her car, and pumped her milk in parking garages between appointments. An airplane pilot pumped and sent her milk back on a return flight while she continued her route.

> 66 To nursing moms who are going back to work: It can be done—I have been back for one month and am pumping 16 ounces a day! 99
>
> —A MOTHER IN AN ONLINE FORUM

Why do they do it? Most mothers choose to pump their milk because they do not wish to give their babies formula instead. A full appreciation of the differences between human milk and manufactured substitutes makes the choice compelling (reread Chapter 2 if you're wavering). Knowing that breast milk, even when delivered in a bottle, is the perfect food for babies' long-term development and health is enough for most women.

For some mothers, the choice to pump rather than to use formula is emotional. "Pumping my milk helps me to keep my work in perspective and my priorities straight," says one woman. "I know that no matter how vexing the rest of my day may be, I'm still accomplishing something worthwhile by giving my milk to my baby."

Pumping your milk is a practical choice during the first months, as it will keep you from becoming uncomfortably full and leaking during the hours you are not with your baby, and reduce your risk of developing plugged ducts and mastitis. Over the months and weeks to come, regular pumping will keep your milk supply plentiful as long as you and your baby continue breastfeeding. (If you will be working 20 hours or more per week, pumping will probably be essential to establishing your milk supply in the first four months.) Pumping will ensure sufficient supplies if your baby has an extra-hungry day while at daycare, or if you need to take an overnight trip or be out on a weekend night. A refrigerator stocked with little bags of frozen breast milk gives a working mother a restful sense of security. All's well, no matter what surprises her day may bring.

In a few lines of work, pumping simply isn't possible. A police detective writes, "I work surveillance from 9:00 P.M. to 5:00 A.M. I'm not alone in the car, and we can't make much noise. Plus, my partner is male. And when I'm not on surveillance, I'm usually in court." But the detective didn't want to wean her baby completely. Having her spouse feed the baby formula during her work hours, and nursing frequently during her off hours, was the only solution for this mother. Once your milk supply is very well established and your baby is interested in eating solid foods as well as nursing, such an arrangement can work for a while. While adding formula to the mix is very likely to decrease your milk supply over time and may lead you to wean earlier than you would otherwise, you can continue to breastfeed even if you absolutely cannot pump. If you must use formula, try to avoid doing so until after the first few months of breastfeeding. Be certain to nurse freely and frequently during weekends, early mornings, evenings, and nights.

You may not need to pump your milk at all if you are returning to work part time. If you are working four hours a day or less, and your baby is four months or older, you may find that she tends to take a long nap while you are gone and wake up hungry only when you return. "I used to leave a bottle of expressed milk with my sitter," says one mother of a five-and-a-half-month-old, "but my daughter seems to prefer just to sleep and wait for me than drink it."

In general, a mother should pump once for every three hours of separation. Your susceptibility to plugged ducts may require you to pump more frequently. If your baby is older, or has begun to "reverse-cycle feed" (see pages 172–74), you may be able to go longer periods without pumping.

Don't allow the prospect of pumping to make you feel you must choose between weaning your baby and giving up your job. Like learning to breastfeed, learning to pump is much easier if you go about it calmly and positively. And, with improvements in the effectiveness and portability of breast pumps, pumping several ounces of milk in a few minutes can be a breeze.

Milk Expression and Supply

The key to a plentiful supply of milk is to drain your breasts frequently and completely, at least seven times every 24 hours. Extended periods of time in which the breasts are not drained decrease milk production. It's a simple system. Levels of prolactin, the milk-making hormone, rise and fall in response to how often and much the breasts are drained.

A gradually falling milk supply sets off a row of dominoes toward weaning. Breasts that go undrained repeatedly over time release substances that act locally in the breast to cause the milk-producing cells to slow or even cease production, further reducing the milk supply. A low milk supply delays the milk let-down response, leading to a frustrated baby, a perplexed mother, and, too often, premature weaning.

A mother may be especially perplexed by this turn of events if she has been pumping her milk every three hours when she's not with her baby. The culprit, most likely, is an inefficient pump that does not drain her breasts sufficiently. Selecting the right method and the best machine for expressing your milk will prevent a gradual reduction in your milk supply and enable you to nurse your baby as long as you both desire.

Hand Expression

For some women, the best method of expressing milk requires no pump at all. Now widely assumed to be difficult and useful only for emergencies, manual expression was once the most common way to collect breast milk. Some mothers still declare that, once they have learned the technique, expressing milk without machinery has become far and away their preferred method. Their choice is quiet, natural, and always available.

Women who do use a pump will find the ability to hand-express useful and a comfort. After all, pump attachments get lost, pumps break, batteries die, and electricity goes out. Some breastfeeding professionals, in addition, believe that hand expression after pumping ensures complete breast drainage and maximizes milk production.

Learning how to hand-express milk takes just a bit of practice. Position your fingers slightly behind and beneath the areola, in the same area that your baby's mouth compresses when he stimulates and drains the breasts. Your thumb and index and middle fingers should be above and below the areola, the thumb at twelve o'clock and your fingers at six o'clock. Use two motions, pushing the thumb backward and then the fingers forward, to press the milk out of the breast. As you continue, rotate the thumb and fingers around the areola. Once you learn the motion, just relax and think of your baby until the milk lets down and flows out.

Some women teach themselves how to perform manual expression while in the shower. The warmth of the water eases the let-down reflex, and spraying milk doesn't make a mess. Another way to begin

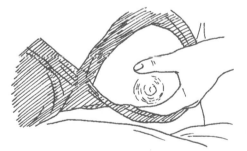

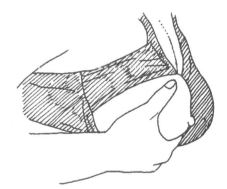

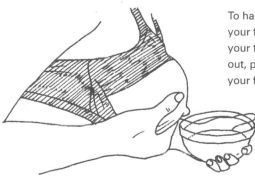

To hand express your milk, place your fingers beneath the areola and your thumb above. To press the milk out, press your thumb backward and your fingers forward.

learning is to experiment on one breast while nursing your baby with the other. With a towel on your lap to catch the spray, you can take advantage of the baby's stimulation to launch a let-down.

HOW TO HAND-EXPRESS YOUR BREAST MILK

1. Wash your hands.

2. Position your thumb and index and middle fingers an inch or two behind the nipple, thumb above, fingers below. (This is the approximate area where the ducts come together beneath the areola.)

3. Push your fingers straight back toward your chest, keeping them the same distance apart. Then gently squeeze them together using a slight rolling motion, lifting the nipple outward. Try not to slide your fingers away from their original position.

4. Relax and think about your baby to hasten your let-down reflex. You can also stimulate your let-down by starting out with a few minutes of breast massage, gently moving your hands toward the nipple. Some mothers find that a minute or two of quick squeezes just behind the nipple mimics a baby's rapid first sucks that set off the let-down.

5. Rotate the fingers around the nipple to help drain the various areas in the breast.

6. Switch back and forth from breast to breast as the flow slows to collect more milk.

After a few sessions, you may well be a master of hand expression, able to drain your breasts and direct a spray of milk into a clean container with ease. Many mothers manage to save time by expressing milk from both breasts simultaneously, using two containers set in front of them on a tabletop. Expect the process, once learned, to take 15 to 20 minutes.

Pumps and Pumping

While mothers have always been able to express milk by using their own hands, pumps designed to extract human milk have been documented from as early as the Victorian era. Throughout the twentieth century, breast pumps were developed and improved upon. The groundbreaking work on electric breast pumps was done in the 1950s by Einar Egnell, whose internal-piston pump remains in use today. Copied by other pump manufacturers, his design is still considered to be the gold standard in breast-pump technology.

Today there are dozens of pumps from which to choose, depending on your needs and circumstances. In all cases, the ideal pump is portable, comfortable, and efficient.

What Makes an Efficient Pump?

Efficiency is the most important quality for a mother who will miss more than one nursing while away from her baby. An efficient pump has an automatic and rapid draw-and-release pattern, repeating 48 to 60 times per minute, about the speed at which a baby nurses. A rapid-cycle breast pump stimulates and drains the breast with nearly the efficiency of a baby, and helps to maintain a plentiful milk supply over the long term. In general, a pump that cycles less frequently will be less successful at stimulating milk let-down and draining the breast.

A slow-cycling pump may seem to work well enough in the early weeks of lactation. As the weeks go by, however, it becomes less able to stimulate the let-down reflex, leading to poor milk drainage and lower milk production. Rarely is the pump pinpointed as the cause; after all, it used to work fine. Instead, a mother may come to believe that she is unable to provide enough milk for her growing baby. Pumps vary in the strength of their suction as well as their speed. Too little suction may be insufficiently stimulating; too much may be painful and inhibit the let-down reflex. Most electric pumps have a dial with which you can adjust the suction to a level that is both comfortable and effective.

Pumps with double-pumping accessory kits, for expressing milk from both breasts simultaneously, stimulate the let-down reflex better and drain the breasts more thoroughly. Double-pumping can also cut the time necessary to express milk in half, a real boon during a busy workday. When double-pumping, mothers report, they can complete a pumping session in 10 to 15 minutes (allowing them to eat lunch or a snack after rather than during pumping). Double pumping may also increase a mother's prolactin levels, and thereby increase her overall milk supply.

A pump's efficiency is also related to the tunnel size of the flange, the attachment that covers the breast. During pumping, the nipple moves back and forth in the tunnel as the pump's suction pulls and releases. Not uncommonly, the tunnel is too small for an individual mother's nipple. When a large nipple (or one enlarged by swelling caused by the suction of the pump), cannot move back and forth in the tunnel, the flow of milk starts to shut down. Pump manufacturers have recently recognized this problem and have begun to produce larger flanges that allow for large nipples to move freely in the tunnel. These larger flanges must be specially ordered.

Choosing the Right Pump for You

The right pump is the one that meets your individual needs. A pump that worked well for a friend or relative may not be appropriate for your schedule, location, body, or budget. Will you need to pump only occasionally, or three times a day, five days a week? Will you be pumping in a private office, a parked car, or at home? How much milk will you need to pump? How much time will you have to pump? How much can you afford to spend on a pump?

> If you work 30 hours a week or more, look for a pump model that includes a double-pumping kit and cycles automatically up to 60 times a minute to avoid a decrease in your milk supply.

The Cost of Pumps

Consider first how long you will be separated from your baby each day. If you expect to need to pump two mornings a week, you probably won't need an expensive hospital-grade electric pump. If you'll be working 40 hours a week or traveling at some point, you will want to invest in, or rent, the best pump you can find.

While cost is certainly a consideration in choosing a pump, keep in mind that if you decide to start out with a less expensive, less efficient pump and find your milk supply dropping, you may need to purchase a second, more efficient pump. Getting the right pump in the first place may actually save you money—especially if it keeps you from switching to formula (most good pumps sold to consumers cost about the same as two months of formula). Automatic pumps may enable you to pump easily while reading, talking on the phone, or eating lunch. They also offer you the valuable option of nearly effortless

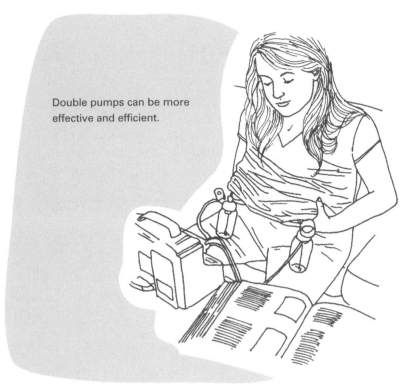

Double pumps can be more effective and efficient.

double-pumping. And you'll be able to reuse a good pump with a second child, if one comes along, more easily than you would a budget pump.

Renting an electric pump from your hospital or from a lactation consultant will save on your initial outlay. If you aren't certain how long you'll be pumping, or if this baby is definitely your last or only baby, renting may be the way to get the best pump for the least money. Over time, though, the rental fees combined with the cost of the accessories kit (the washable flanges, bottles, and tubing that come in contact with your breasts and milk) may cost more than a good new pump.

If you are considering borrowing a pump from a friend or purchasing a secondhand electric pump, be aware that many breast pumps are approved by the U.S. Food and Drug Administration (FDA) as "single user" equipment, not to be shared or resold. Pumps can't always be adequately sterilized, and it is possible, if they are reused, for certain viruses to be transmitted from woman to woman. Even with a new accessories kit, airborne pathogens can enter the pump motor and put the next user at risk. (One pump, the Hollister Purely Yours, is supposed to be incapable of spreading airborne germs, although the FDA designates it, too, for single users.) Another problem with borrowed and secondhand pumps, say pump manufacturers, is that older electric pumps may lose some speed and suction over time. (Rental pumps are classified as multi-user, because they have barriers to keep milk out of the motors.)

Mothers who qualify for the Special Supplemental Nutrition Program for Women, Infants, and Children (WIC) and who work or attend school are eligible for the loan of a portable electric pump. To locate a WIC office near your home, look for a listing in the phone book or contact your county or city health department. Medela and Hollister, two large pump manufacturers, offer a limited number of free or reduced-cost pumps to mothers with financial need. Mothers who do not qualify for WIC, and yet find the cost of an electric pump beyond their means, may find local lactation consultants and other rental-pump providers open to discussing various payment options.

Pump Design

Although many pumps are on the market, a few general designs have proven effective, depending on a mother's needs and circumstances.

HAND-OPERATED PUMPS

If you plan to work no more than three hours a day or mostly at home, you may want to consider a manual pump. Easy to wash and carry, manuals can work well for women who don't want to lug anything that can't be fit into a handbag. Students who already must carry a load of books around often choose manuals because they are small and light and quiet, and do not need an electrical outlet to run (though pumps that run on batteries can also save the search for an outlet). Hand pumps are best for occasional use, as they express milk from only one side at a time, and it is difficult to make them work at the speed with which a baby sucks. Also, the flange size may be too small for large nipples. Still, if you use an electric pump it is wise to have a hand-operated pump in the house as a backup in case the power goes out (learning to express your milk manually is also a useful backup plan). Among the best manual pumps are Avent's Isis pump and Medela's Harmony pump.

INEXPENSIVE PERSONAL-USE ELECTRIC PUMPS

Usually available for less than $200, these are also recommended for occasional use only. They run on power from an electrical outlet, batteries, or, in some cases, either. Many of the pumps in this category are, frankly, a waste of money. If they are "semi-automatic," you will need to use a finger to create the draw-and-release suction pattern. Although a few of these pumps enable double pumping (pumping both breasts simultaneously), most cycle slowly, too slowly to drain a breast effectively. Many of these pumps are less effective than skillful hand expression. Exceptions include Medela's Single Deluxe and the Nurture III electric pump.

HIGH-END PERSONAL-USE ELECTRIC PUMPS

Pumps in this category are lightweight and portable and run on electricity from either a battery pack or an outlet. Since most have automatic draw-and-release suction and cycle at least the necessary minimum of 48 times per minute, they are a good choice for mothers who will be working more than 20 hours each week. If you will be working 30 hours a week or more, look for models that cycle up to 60 times a minute, to avoid a decrease in your milk supply. These pumps usually come with attractive, briefcase- or backpack-style carrying cases and all of the parts necessary to pump one or both breasts simultaneously. The cost, at this writing, ranges from $180 to $350. Make sure the pump you choose comes with a full-year warranty.

WHICH PUMP DO YOU NEED?

If you work less than 20 hours a week:

> None (express manually instead)
>
> Hand pump
>
> Inexpensive battery-operated pump

If you work more than 20 hours a week:

> Personal-use electric pump
>
> Rental pump

If you are a student or have a variable schedule:

> None (express manually instead)
>
> Personal-use electric pump
>
> Rental pump with battery option

If you travel without your baby:

> Personal-use electric pump
>
> Rental pump with battery option

Popular choices in this category are Medela's Pump In Style and Hollister's Purely Yours.

RENTAL ELECTRIC PUMPS

Generally too expensive for individuals to buy, these highly efficient pumps are designed for multiple users and are widely available to rent. Fully automatic, with a speed of 48 to 60 cycles a minute, most are lightweight and portable, and they run on battery packs when electrical outlets aren't available. Rental rates vary around the country, so you will want to shop around. You may be able to rent at a discount if you commit to a rental period of three to six months. You'll also need to purchase an accessories kit for personal use. Kits are available for double pumping for around $50. The leading pumps in this category are Medela's Lactina and Hollister's Elite.

NEW-TECHNOLOGY PUMPS

These newer pumps are available both for purchase and to rent. Two of these pumps use two distinct sucking patterns: The first imitates the initial light, fast sucking an infant does to elicit the let-down response; the second sucks longer and deeper, as a baby does once the milk begins to flow. Another new pump is a shield-shaped device, similar to the breast shells that are used to protect sore nipples or pull out inverted nipples; it is placed inside the bra and cycles automatically and hands-free. Another uses very low constant suction with a soft cup that expresses the milk into a flat plastic bag. Designed to keep your hands free to write or do other tasks as you pump, these pumps have received mixed reviews from mothers and lactation consultants. Two new-technology pumps that are gaining fans are Medela's Symphony (a rental) and Medela's Pump In Style Advanced (a personal-use pump).

Whichever model you select, the bottom line on choosing a pump is that the best come with a one-year warranty, cycle at least 48 times per minute, and are recommended, sold, or rented by lactation consultants. Avoid pumps that are sold in drug or discount stores, that are not labeled with the number of cycles per minutes, or that do not come with a warranty.

Other Supplies for Expressing Milk

Unless you use a pump that comes with an insulated cooler compartment, like the Pump in Style or Purely Yours, you will need something in which to transport your expressed milk. Several coolers designed for the purpose are now available through catalogs, maternity shops, and baby-supply stores. These coolers, which come with freezer packs, will keep as much as 36 ounces of milk cold in the refrigerator for up to 16 hours. Some of the coolers double as pump carriers. If you'll be leaving your pump at work or hand-expressing, though, you may want a cooler designed to carry just milk and bottles. A less expensive and perfectly satisfactory alternative is a lunch bag with a freezer pack or large-mouthed thermal bottle filled a third of the way with crushed ice. Tuck in a sealed milk bag full of fresh breast milk, and it will stay well cooled until you are home or at the caregiver's.

If you'll be plugging your pump into a wall socket, you may wish to add a 10- to 12-foot extension cord and a three-prong adapter to your pump carrier, if space allows, so that you'll have more flexibility in where you can pump. Other useful items you might include in your pump tote are extra bottle lids, rubber bands, freezer tape, a hand towel, and, in case the power goes out, a backup manual pump.

Getting to Know Your Pump

Wait until your baby is at least two weeks old before trying out your breast pump. Until then, although you may be overflowing with milk and letting down continually (when you're nursing and when you're not), you need to focus on learning to breastfeed your baby. Establishing a bountiful milk supply and becoming comfortable with breastfeeding will promote successful pumping far better than will getting an early start on pumping.

It feels odd to hook yourself up to a machine. Even though the newest pumps are easy to use, you will want to spend some time getting comfortable with your pump, so that you can relax as you use it, and thereby obtain more milk in less time. If you must return to work just six weeks after your baby's birth, begin practicing with your breast pump between two and four weeks after birth. Be sure to store any of the milk you obtain rather than giving it to your baby. At this age she still needs to breastfeed exclusively to become an expert nurser as well as to keep up your prolactin levels and to establish your milk supply. Some time between the second and fourth week, you can begin to accustom your baby to a bottle (see Introducing the Bottle, page 159).

Relaxation promotes a speedy let-down even with a less effective pump. Begin any pumping session with a routine that will help you relax and feel comfortable. A good time to pump is the early morning, when your milk supply is most plentiful and you are probably more relaxed than at the end of the day. Pump soon after feeding your baby. (If your baby has taken only one breast, you should be able to collect enough milk to store.) If you are using a pump that requires only one hand, you can pump while simultaneously nursing your baby; your milk will let down very quickly this way.

First wash your hands. Choose a comfortable chair near a table where you can set your pump and bottles. Set up the pump following the manufacturer's instructions. Expose both your breasts (you'll learn to pump with less exposure later). Lightly massage your breasts with your fingertips in small circular patterns to stimulate your let-down reflex. Holding a warm (not hot) heating pad against your breasts can help, too. Looking at your baby, imagining her, or sniffing a piece of clothing she has recently worn may also speed the let-down of your milk. Soon pumping will require less preparation, but in the beginning it is helpful to spend some time in preparing your mind as well as your machinery.

Bring the flange of the pump against your breast so that your nipple is centered in the opening. (If you have very large nipples and are using an electric pump, you can buy a special flange from the pump manufacturer. Ask the lactation consultant or La Leche League leader who runs your rental station about this.) You may wish to dampen the flange to create a stronger seal between it and your breast. Turn an automatic pump to its lowest setting, or begin to manually pump in a slow, gentle rhythm. Gradually increase the speed. If pumping is painful, the suction may be too strong, or your

GERRY ANNE'S RECIPE FOR
PUMPING SUCCESS

(From Gerry Anne Dubis, a La Leche League leader)

Before beginning your pumping career, it is important to understand two things:

1. Morning pumpings will yield the most milk, whether you're pumping at home or at work.

2. The amount of milk yielded will probably decline with each pumping as the day goes on.

Begin to pump this way:

1. Nurse the baby well on one side between 5:00 A.M. and 8:00 A.M. Pump the other side for approximately 10 minutes. Then nurse the baby on the pumped side to further drain the breast.

2. Refrigerate or freeze the milk.

3. Later in the morning, about one and a half hours after a feeding or during the baby's nap, pump both breasts.

4. Chill this milk, add it to the milk already refrigerated, and then freeze the container. If you froze the milk you collected earlier, freeze this portion separately, or chill it before adding it to the frozen milk. (Do not add warm milk to chilled or frozen milk.)

5. You have finished pumping for the day. For the rest of the day, just take care of yourself and your baby.

Assuming you collect 3 to 4 ounces of milk per day, pumping twice a day for three weeks will put 63 to 84 ounces of milk in your freezer before you return to work. With practice, you may soon be able to pump as much as 8 ounces in a day. At that rate, in three weeks you can collect 164 ounces!

nipple may be positioned incorrectly. A good pump should not cause discomfort.

With practice, you should be able to drain both breasts in 10 to 15 minutes if you're using a fully automatic pump with a double collection kit, 20 to 30 minutes otherwise. In general, pumping should take only as long as it takes to nurse your baby.

Save any milk you collect (see Collecting Milk for Storage, page 155). Every 2 to 3 ounces is another bag of gold in your freezer. To increase your stock of frozen milk, you might grab your pump after any feeding when the baby has taken only one breast.

Another trick for maximizing your milk collecting, if you are using a single-side pump, is to switch back and forth between your breasts every few minutes as the flow slows. Pumping both sides at once is even more effective for increasing milk output.

Care and Handling of Expressed Breast Milk

Breast milk is a highly stable substance; that is, it doesn't go bad easily. (Formula, on the other hand, is an unstable substance that spoils quickly.) Teeming with white cells scouring it for viruses and other pathogens, fresh breast milk protects itself from contamination just as it protects your baby from infection. It can be kept safe and ready for your baby for varying periods of time, depending on how it is handled and the temperature at which it is stored. Chilled fresh breast milk will retain almost all of its immunological properties for 72 hours.

Even short-term lack of refrigeration isn't a problem. One small study (of 8 to 10 samples) found that freshly expressed milk could be kept at room temperature for up to 10 hours without spoiling. Those white cells just keep doing their job. To be on the safe side, however, most mothers keep their fresh milk chilled in a small cooler with freezer packs when refrigeration isn't available.

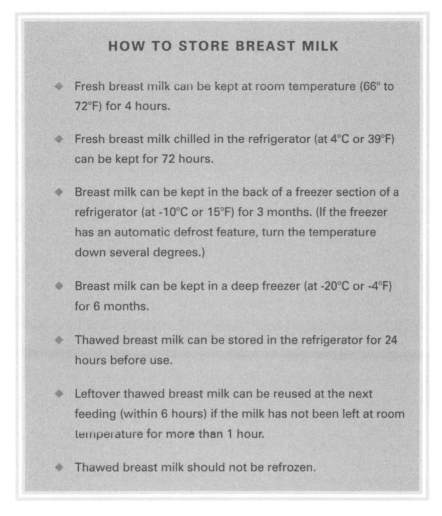

HOW TO STORE BREAST MILK

◆ Fresh breast milk can be kept at room temperature (66° to 72°F) for 4 hours.

◆ Fresh breast milk chilled in the refrigerator (at 4°C or 39°F) can be kept for 72 hours.

◆ Breast milk can be kept in the back of a freezer section of a refrigerator (at -10°C or 15°F) for 3 months. (If the freezer has an automatic defrost feature, turn the temperature down several degrees.)

◆ Breast milk can be kept in a deep freezer (at -20°C or -4°F) for 6 months.

◆ Thawed breast milk can be stored in the refrigerator for 24 hours before use.

◆ Leftover thawed breast milk can be reused at the next feeding (within 6 hours) if the milk has not been left at room temperature for more than 1 hour.

◆ Thawed breast milk should not be refrozen.

Freezing inactivates the white blood cells in breast milk. It does not, however, affect the many other antimicrobial properties of breast milk, which inhibit the growth of bacteria when the milk is-handled and stored properly. Freezing doesn't affect any of the known nutrients in breast milk.

You can help those busy white cells keep your milk clean and ready to use in several ways. Always wash your hands before expressing your milk. Store your milk in disposable containers designed for the purpose or in tightly closed containers that have been washed with hot soapy water, rinsed, and left to air-dry. Label your containers with the date the milk was collected, and use the oldest stored milk first. Don't store your milk in the door of your freezer; the temperature there fluctuates a lot when the freezer is opened and closed. Store it instead in the back of the refrigerator freezer, where the temperature is constant, or better yet, in a deep freezer.

Color, Scent, and Taste

Depending on the foods a mother eats or the medications she may be taking, expressed breast milk can be a pale hue of almost any color, from creamy white to the palest blue. Vegetarian mothers who eat loads of salad may have greenish milk. Moms fond of tomato sauce on their pasta may have pinkish milk. All pale shades are normal, and none indicates that the milk has spoiled.

Milk that has been stored for a couple of hours may look oddly layered. The high-fat hindmilk, the cream, rises to the top, as it does in any mammal's milk. This, too, is perfectly normal and not a sign of spoilage. Gently shake the milk to reblend the fat. The amount of fat you see varies depending on when the milk was pumped. Milk pumped right after nursing the baby will have a higher percentage of fat than if it were pumped just before a feeding.

Fresh breast milk has a mild, sweet scent and taste. It also echoes the flavors and scents of a mother's diet, as it does the colors of the foods she eats. If a woman is eating, in general, the same foods during lactation that she ate during pregnancy, the unique flavor of her breast milk is already familiar to and favored by her baby. Fetal taste buds are formed and functioning by 13 to 15 weeks' gestation. From that point forward, researchers believe, fetuses sip amniotic fluid. (They even gulp it, causing hiccups from time to time.) Like breast milk, amniotic fluid carries the dominant flavors of a mother's diet, such as curry, garlic, or onions. After birth, the newborn begins to nurse and enjoys the already familiar flavors of his mother's diet through her breast milk. When he begins to sample solids, he will accept with pleasure a bit of curry or a nibble of beans and rice, if that's what his mother has often eaten. It's a nifty way in which nature acclimates babies, beginning in the womb, to the menus of the culture into which they are born.

Sometimes breast milk develops a slightly soapy smell and taste after it has been chilled or frozen. This alteration is thought to be caused by the fat-digesting enzyme lipase as it becomes active. A few infants will object to it; most won't care a bit. If your baby accepts fresh milk without a murmur but rejects milk that has been stored, try heating your fresh milk in a pan on the stove to the point just before boiling (scalding, in culinary lingo) before freezing it for later use. Doing so will halt the process of fat digestion and prevent a soapy smell or taste. Scalding will inactivate some of the nutrients, including Vitamin C, but many will remain.

Collecting Milk for Storage

You may find yourself sometimes collecting small amounts, just an ounce or two, of milk, especially when you first start using your pump. You can freeze these small portions separately, and thaw several at once for your baby's meals. Or you can combine small portions of milk in the refrigerator or freezer. Be sure to chill newly expressed milk before adding it to chilled or frozen milk. Doing so keeps the older milk from being re-warmed by the new milk, which could possibly lead to spoilage.

There is some controversy about which containers are best for storing breast milk, fresh or frozen. The possibilities include glass, polycarbonate (clear) plastic, and polypropylene (cloudy) plastic bottles or other containers. It is thought that some white cells in breast milk will cling to glass, although they release after the milk has been stored for a couple of hours. For healthy breastfed babies who get most of their milk from Mom, and only a portion from bottles, this potential loss of a few white cells isn't a concern. Although plastic containers are more easily obtained these days, some lactation consultants prefer glass. They are concerned that bisphenol, a common plasticizer in polycarbonate bottles and a possible carcinogen, may leach into milk. You might instead choose cloudy or colored polypropylene containers designed specifically for breast-milk storage, or select from the array of general-purpose food-storage containers in the supermarket.

Plastic milk-storage bags are also popular. They come pre-sterilized and have a space on which to write the collection date. Disposable bottle liners, which are less expensive, can also be used for freezing milk, but they are thinner than milk storage bags and more likely to split at the seams during freezing and leak during defrosting. Plastic bags of either type take up less space in a freezer than bottles or other rigid containers. Bags, however, are not reusable, and it's difficult to add fresh milk to an already sealed and frozen bag of milk. Unlike bottles, bags can't be used for feeding thawed milk directly to a baby.

When pouring fresh milk into a bag or other container, be sure to leave space at the top for the milk to expand into as it freezes.

To seal a bag, roll it down to about an inch above the milk, and close it with a bit of freezer tape. Or twist the top of the bag, bend the top down, and seal the bag with a rubber band or a wire twist tie; it will be easier to open this way. Write the date on the tape that seals the bag, on a separate piece of tape, or on the label provided for this purpose. To keep your milk bags from getting jostled, punctured, or buried in the freezer, you might place them upright in a heavy plastic container.

One storage system, Milk Mates, includes 10 polypropylene bottles with lids and a rack that allows the milk to be stored sideways, saving freezer space. The rolling rack dispenses the bottles in order of collection date, oldest milk first.

Using Stored Milk

You may find that on most working days you never need to freeze your milk at all. You drop the day's output at pick-up time with your daycare provider for your baby's lunch the next day. Occasionally, you'll need more milk than you've pumped, because your baby is extra hungry, you're going out for the evening, or you missed a pumping session. Then your stored supplies of frozen milk prove their worth.

When you need to break into your frozen milk supplies, take out the oldest milk first to avoid having to throw out outdated milk. Thaw the milk quickly by holding the bag under warm running water or swirling it in a bowl of warm water, or thaw it over several hours in the refrigerator. Milk thawed in the refrigerator must be used within 24 hours of placing it there, and it should not be re-frozen. Do not thaw milk by letting it sit at room temperature.

Refrigerated fresh milk, your daycare provider will be glad to know, simply needs to have the chill taken off by running it under warm (not hot) water or placing it in a bowl of warm water or in a bottle warmer. It should not be heated until it is hot; that would destroy some of its immunological properties.

Breast milk should never be thawed or heated in a microwave oven. The high heat produced by microwaves can destroy the immunological properties and many of the nutrients in breast milk. In addition, the uneven heating of microwaves, even those with turntables, may partially melt plastic bottles and other plastic containers, releasing chemicals into the milk.

When frozen breast milk thaws, the fat in the milk separates and rises to the top. Gently shaking the bottle will blend the fat back in with the rest of the milk.

What happens if you thaw a few ounces of breast milk and your baby takes only half of it? What do you do with the leftover milk? Although laboratory research is lacking in this area, most lactation consultants believe that thawed or even warmed milk can be safely refrigerated, re-warmed, and used for the next feeding, as long as it has not been left at room temperature for longer than one hour.

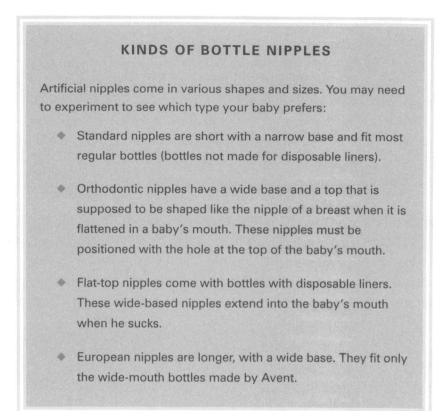

KINDS OF BOTTLE NIPPLES

Artificial nipples come in various shapes and sizes. You may need to experiment to see which type your baby prefers:

◆ Standard nipples are short with a narrow base and fit most regular bottles (bottles not made for disposable liners).

◆ Orthodontic nipples have a wide base and a top that is supposed to be shaped like the nipple of a breast when it is flattened in a baby's mouth. These nipples must be positioned with the hole at the top of the baby's mouth.

◆ Flat-top nipples come with bottles with disposable liners. These wide-based nipples extend into the baby's mouth when he sucks.

◆ European nipples are longer, with a wide base. They fit only the wide-mouth bottles made by Avent.

Feeding Expressed Milk

Babies younger than six months are most often fed expressed milk in a bottle with a rubber or silicone nipple. Most babies are able to begin drinking from a cup at six months of age, although many continue using a bottle through the first year, and sometimes beyond.

As with pumps and storage containers, you have several choices in bottle model depending on your needs and circumstances and your baby's own mysterious preferences. The best bottles are easy to clean and have accurate measuring indicators. Bottles molded into unusual shapes or split down the middle for self-feeding are nearly impossible to clean. Angled bottles are supposed to make it easier to keep the nipple filled, but this is just as easy to do with straight bottles. Some bottles come with disposable liners, which are supposed to cause less air swallowing. They don't. The disposable bags are sterilized, but sterilization is unnecessary when feeding breast milk because it handles germ control on its own. All in all, the extra cost of a feeding system that uses disposable bags probably outweighs any benefits.

The Adiri Breastbottle Nurser is an interesting innovation. Made of soft, translucent silicone and shaped like a breast, it may be easier for some babies to latch on to than standard bottles, although it is a little harder for an adult to hold. Sold by online vendors, it also allows the baby or adult to better control the flow of milk, by pressing on the soft, pliable side of the bottle.

Most bottles come in both 4-ounce and 8-ounce sizes. Four-ounce bottles make more sense for babies who take only 2 to 4 ounces at a feeding. Eight-ounce bottles will come in handy later, when your baby drinks 5 to 6 ounces at a feeding.

Artificial nipples are made of latex rubber or silicone. Silicone nipples are preferred, as rubber has a taste and odor and deteriorates faster than silicone. Rubber is also harder to clean and so should be washed by hand, rather than in a dishwasher.

Nipples come in various shapes and flow speeds. Your choice of nipples will be limited somewhat by your choice of bottles. If possible, try a few different nipples; babies sometimes reject all but one shape of nipple, although that shape varies from baby to baby.

Introducing the Bottle

While a lot of babies are able to switch back and forth between Mom's breast and an artificial nipple (especially if it's not Mom who is offering the substitute), a few babies object to anything but the real thing. To avert protests, introduce a bottle as soon as breastfeeding is well established. A bottle can be introduced between two and four weeks of age, as long as the baby is latching on to the breast well. Waiting longer than a month may result in lack of cooperation on the part of the baby.

You can begin to learn to use your pump at the same time, expressing an ounce or two here and there. If you feel your milk begin to let down when you're not nursing the baby, and you have a free hand, grab your pump and collect the milk that's on its way. Store these harvested ounces in the freezer, or use them fresh as you introduce a bottle to your baby.

Don't introduce a bottle by using formula rather than breast milk. Formula tastes quite different from breast milk, and a baby may refuse the bottle on taste alone. You want your baby to bridge the difference of nursing on an artificial nipple, only to discover that familiar, sweet breast milk waits for him on the other side.

You can give your baby a try at the bottle during the late afternoon, when many new moms feel a little depleted anyway, or when your partner or a relative is around and you'd like to go out for a walk. An ounce or two of milk is enough to give the baby some practice at this new sort of sucking.

Give the baby a practice session every two to three days. Sometimes, once a baby has taken a bottle, we assume that he will always take it and stop offering it for practice sessions. Babies may have other ideas, however, and change their minds. Offer the bottle regularly to maintain his acceptance.

When offering a bottle to a baby, you may wish to ask your partner or another caregiver to try first. Often a baby will happily accept a substitute feeding from someone other than Mom, especially if Mom is out of the room, out of earshot, and cannot even be smelled by baby. Be sure then to offer the bottle in a location other than Mom and baby's favorite nursing chair, which may carry the scent of her body and milk. (On the other hand, some parents report success with wrapping the baby in a blouse or nightgown his mother has recently worn while offering the bottle.)

Getting a baby to take a bottle should not be a contest of wills, but gentle persuasion. End the practice session if either baby or caregiver feels upset. Try a couple of times each day, both when the baby seems hungry and when he is not, when he is asleep and when he is alert, at home and away from home, and with Mom and with another caregiver.

You can begin in several ways. You or your helper should hold the baby in your arms just as you do when you're nursing. Wait for the baby to open his mouth rather than pushing in the nipple. Many babies willingly take the bottle when they are given the breast for a few minutes and then their mother quickly slips in the bottle. Some babies are much more willing to take a bottle when placed in a forward-facing position, back against your chest, legs facing forward. Holding the bottle in the baby's mouth with one hand while patting his bottom with the other, while walking around the room, sometimes does the trick. Placing the baby in a sling may help keep your hands free to hold the bottle and pat his bottom. Some babies will take a bottle while being swayed from side to side. Some babies will take a bottle when they are riding in a car seat. Once a baby becomes accustomed to taking a bottle in one place he is more likely to drink from it in other places.

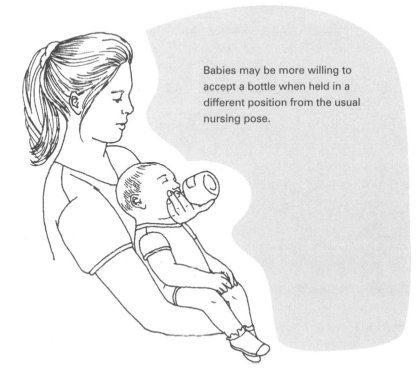

Babies may be more willing to accept a bottle when held in a different position from the usual nursing pose.

Keep in mind that some babies will take a bottle from their care-givers at daycare when they won't from anybody at home. These babies seem to be thinking, "I'm not at home, so I don't eat the way I do at home." Of course, many caregivers have years of experience helping babies to feel at ease in new situations, and can perform apparent miracles.

Once the baby begins to suck on the nipple, be patient when he pauses; don't urge him to suck continuously. Let him control the rate of his feeding, just as he does when he nurses. If the baby signals that he has had enough at any point, let him end the meal, even if there is breast milk left in the bottle.

A full feeding of 3 to 4 ounces of breast milk should take about 5 to 15 minutes, once the baby gets going. (You may wish to put just an ounce or so in the bottle for the very first feedings, to avoid wasting any breast milk.) Full feedings that require longer than 15 minutes may be due to slow flow from a nipple that is plugged or has too small a hole. A sign that nipple flow may be too fast is a sputtering baby who pulls off frequently.

If the baby seems resistant at first, and refuses the bottle, consider first the nipple you are using. Try another shape, particularly if the nipple flow seems slow. Do not allow these sessions to become too upsetting for the baby or yourself.

Occasionally, a baby will refuse all bottles, regardless of timing, caregiver, bottle, or nipple shape. If you're faced with a baby who cannot be persuaded, bless his firm little heart, try a few creative maneuvers. If your baby is older than eight weeks and is handling and mouthing teething rings and other toys, you may wish to add a plastic bottle with a nipple to his toy collection. He will naturally explore it with his mouth. At some point you may wish to put an ounce of breast milk in the bottle and see what happens. Some babies prefer a warm, soft nipple (sound familiar?), so you might warm the bottle nipple under warm running tap water before offering it. If your baby is teething, you might try cooling the bottle nipple in the refrigerator to soothe his gums.

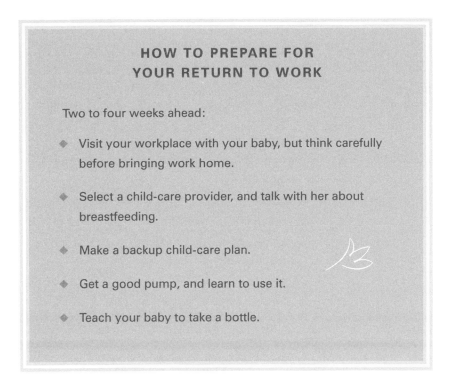

HOW TO PREPARE FOR
YOUR RETURN TO WORK

Two to four weeks ahead:

- Visit your workplace with your baby, but think carefully before bringing work home.

- Select a child-care provider, and talk with her about breastfeeding.

- Make a backup child-care plan.

- Get a good pump, and learn to use it.

- Teach your baby to take a bottle.

Above all, don't panic. Your baby's dismissal of artificial nipples does not mean you cannot return to work. You can forgo bottles altogether, after all. If your baby is four or five months old when you return to work, you may prefer that he be fed from a cup in any case, so that you don't need to wean him from a bottle later. Even babies as young as eight weeks can be fed from a cup; Medela and Ameda/Egnell make soft feeding cups for very young babies. Babies have also been successfully fed with spoons and eyedroppers when their mothers aren't there to nurse them. Talk to a lactation consultant about a bottle-free method that may work for your baby.

If your baby takes a bottle easily, firmly establish the nursing, working mother's rule: "My baby gets a bottle when I'm not there, and breastfeeds when I am there." Your breasts need the stimulation of your nursing baby during your off-hours to maintain and build your milk supply.

seven

YOUR RETURN TO THE OUTSIDE WORLD

"Everybody expects me to be the same person. But I'm a different person."

YOUR FIRST DAYS BACK AT WORK can feel like a visit to your old high school a year after you've graduated. You speak the language, and people may recognize you, but you feel very far removed. Give yourself time; the strangeness will fade.

Although these first weeks will pass quickly, they can be physically and emotionally draining. You may feel just as spent and fragile as you did in the first weeks after the baby was born, but now you must be on your feet and doing things all day. Your emotions may be as strong as during those newborn days—and taxing your energy reserves as much as any physical demands. Not only are you adjusting to being separated from your baby for hours at a time, but your old life and your new life stand face to face—and you must find a way to blend them into one. On top of these challenges, when you go back to work other people assume that everything is back to "normal," and that you are ready to carry on in all ways just as you did before the baby was born. You may be making that assumption yourself.

Now as in the newborn days, you need to take especially good care of yourself. Now as then, you need to reach out to your sources of support. Phone working friends with babies for encouragement, and talk with colleagues who have treaded this path. Consider asking a helpful relative, if you haven't already, to stay with you now for a week or more. Accept offers of assistance from friends and neighbors, although such offers may not be as plentiful as just after birth. Be sure that your partner, especially, does not assume that the end of your maternity leave means that now everything is (at last) as it was before. You will need his help and understanding more than anything else.

Take care, however, when you seek advice and assistance. People tend to hold strong beliefs about what is right for mothers and babies. Some people in your life may feel adamantly that you should not work out of the house once you have a baby. Or they may believe that you should "get over it" and, putting the emotions of new motherhood behind you, not let having a baby change you in any way. Filtering out their prejudices might be easy if you were sure of your own feelings. But at the moment you, like most mothers at this juncture, may be fluctuating from confidence to confusion by the hour. You need to figure out what is right for you and your baby, and you need time in which to do it. Someone else's experience or beliefs, and any advice based on them, need not be a factor in your decision making. Welcome encouragement and information, not persuasion.

Combating Fatigue

Regardless of the duties you are now re-shouldering, your first responsibility is to stay as rested as possible. Luckily breastfeeding requires that you sit or lie down and relax several times a day, while accomplishing something important—feeding the baby. Even pumping, once you are comfortable with it, builds in at least two "time-outs" during your day in which you can immerse yourself in a pool of calm and purposeful idleness. Be sure that you get to bed as early as possible every night. Save errands for the weekend, and then do only the bare essentials. Skip doing all but the most necessary household cleaning and other chores for now. In short, you still need to take tender care of yourself. Not only do you deserve it, but staying rested is essential to avoiding plugged breast ducts and infections.

> A really helpful baby gift: a cleaning service for your first weeks back at work.

Bringing your baby into your room to sleep, if you have not already done so, can be a big help. This can save you from getting up or even waking completely several times a night. Keeping your baby near you at night can give you and your baby as much as seven to eight additional hours of physical contact each day. Having your baby within arm's reach means you'll nurse more often at night, guaranteeing a bountiful milk supply. If you prefer not to have your baby sleep in your bed, drop one side of his crib and push the crib up against your bed. You can then reach over and bring your baby beside you to nurse and put him back without ever getting up. (Bolt the crib to the bed, if necessary, so that your baby cannot slip into the crack between the two.) "Sidecar" cribs designed for this purpose are also available.

You might put your baby down for the night in his own bed (in your room or his), and, after he wakes for his first nursing, bring him to your room for the rest of the night. This way he gets accustomed to sleeping in his own bed, so that a full transition may be easier when he is weaned and when you and your partner want your room back to yourselves.

Many mothers report that middle-of-the-night nursings are their favorite times. It's so quiet and peaceful, and you and your baby seem like the only people on earth. No one else needs you, there's nowhere to go; you can just be together.

If you find that you get less rest rather than more with your baby in your room, you might have him spend the night in his crib but bring him into your bed to nurse when he wakes at about five or six o'clock in the morning. This way you can have a long cuddle, perhaps dozing for another hour or two, and your baby's day will begin with a good, long dose of Mom and her milk. You might also put a twin bed in the baby's room and use it to nurse on while lying down.

Nursing provides another essential rest stop at the end of your working day. Nurse your baby as soon as you arrive at the sitter's house or the daycare center. See how he wriggles when he hears your voice, how he relaxes his body against your own and turns to nurse with comical determination. He needs this, and so do you. As soon as you are home, get a snack and a large glass of water or juice, and sit down for a long cuddle and a nursing. Better yet, lie down on the sofa and take a nap while your baby nurses.

If you have older children, you might give them a snack and spread a large quilt on the living room floor for a daily rest and cuddle hour instead of launching right into the usual dinnertime frenzy. Like your baby, your older children are more likely to play happily while you prepare dinner if they've had their time with you first. You may want to hire a neighborhood teenager to come over every afternoon and evening to help get dinner started and to do a load of laundry or two so that you can focus on your children.

Take life slowly on weekends. Afternoon naps and early bedtimes on Saturdays and Sundays should be the rule for the first six months of nursing and working. At any time of day, nursing while lying down and napping is a perfect way to nurture your baby while getting the rest you need. Don't begin any major home improvement projects or restart your social life with a vengeance just yet. The time will come again when you can drive yourself harder. Right now you need to reserve your energy for taking care of yourself and your baby.

Pay careful attention to the quality of your diet now, too, just as you did in the early weeks after birth. You need nutritious, high-protein snacks both at home and at the office, and lots of fluids. Limit the amount of fat in your diet, however, because too much can cause chronic plugged ducts.

Keep a bag of trail mix in your desk at work, and a squeeze bottle of water close at hand all day long.

Exercise will help you combat fatigue, too. You may feel too short on time and energy right now to sign up for aerobics classes, but a regular evening walk (with or without your baby) will help you sleep more restfully and give you more energy.

How Your Baby Adjusts

Sometimes we forget to take care of ourselves because we are so concerned with how our babies are faring. How will your baby adjust to your return to work? The stronger your attachment, the more easily baby will adjust, reveals recent research. Reviewing the data from a large, long-term study of more than 1,000 children from birth through age 8, the National Institute of Child Health and Human Development (NICHHD) has identified the quality of the infant-mother attachment as the single element that enables a baby to thrive in daycare and avoid developmental difficulties down the road. The NICHHD researchers conclude, "A baby's attachment to her mother is the best measure of her social and emotional well-being."

Because you are a responsive mother who has learned to read your baby's cues, your intuition will be your best guide to how well your baby is managing. How does your baby *seem* after a couple of weeks or more of daycare? Is she fussier and clingier than before? Or does she seem like her same wonderful self? Another sign to look for is a developing attachment between your baby and your sitter. Are they becoming truly fond of each other? If so, terrific! You have enlarged your baby's emotional world to include another consistently present, nurturing adult caregiver.

One sign that your baby may not be settling in at daycare is end-of-day reports from the caregiver on behavior that just doesn't sound like your baby's. Consistently unfamiliar behavior may be a sign that your sitter and your baby are not developing a comfortable relationship and that your baby may need another kind of care. One mother who began taking her baby to family daycare when she was eight months old found that her usually merry baby sobbed all day every day until pickup time. At eight months, often a time of intense separation anxiety, this baby simply couldn't adjust to daycare away from home. Her mother found a sitter who could come to her house for a few months, and the baby was able to adjust better. When the baby turned a year old, the mother tried family daycare again, and this time the baby settled in happily.

Babies often become fussy and sensitive the moment their mothers arrive at daycare after work. The provider may interject at this moment that the baby "hasn't cried all day," unintentionally implying that she is in tears because her mother has come. In a way, the implication is correct. Babies often wait until they are with their mothers to express all the frustrations and other feelings that have built up during the day. They know they are with the one person who can meet all their needs, and therefore they feel free to express them. School-age children do the same thing. If your reunions after work are marked by fussiness and crying, it's because your baby has saved a day's worth of her expressions of need for the person who really matters—you.

Take care not to interpret normal developmental changes as signs that your attachment is being disrupted. Working mothers, along with the rest of society, tend to blame everything that goes wrong with their children on the fact that their mothers work. Understanding what your child is likely to do whether you are working or not can keep you from being hard on yourself. The fact is that most infant behavior is unrelated to the mother's employment and unaffected by it, *if* the mother and baby are well attached.

At three to four months, for example, babies suddenly notice how fascinating the world is. Sometimes nursing a baby at this distractible age can seem more like a wrestling match as your baby wiggles and turns his head away because he can't bear to miss what else is going on (babies with exciting siblings are especially prone to this behavior). Although this developmental stage will soon pass—a five- to six-month-old baby will nurse with more resolve—it often coincides with a mother's return to work, and she may take it as a sign that her baby is somehow rejecting her.

On rare occasions, likewise, babies will stage "nursing strikes" during which they refuse the breast completely. Nursing strikes can have a range of causes: Something in the mother's diet may be making her milk taste different or causing an allergic reaction, the baby's gums may ache from teething, he may have a thrush infection, the mother's milk supply may be low, or the milk may be slow to let down. All these problems are correctable, and usually a striking baby can be coaxed back onto the breast. Nevertheless, a working mother may mistakenly and painfully interpret her baby's pushing and turning away during nursings—or sudden refusal to nurse at all—as a rejection.

Teething also can be a source of stress for mother and baby. A baby can cut teeth at four months or even earlier, and experience all the side effects that may come along with teething—fussiness, drooling, chewing, appetite loss, and restless nights—for weeks before a tooth comes in. If such behavior coincides with your return to work, consider teething as a possible reason.

Separation anxiety also gives working mothers angst. Peaking at any time between eight and eighteen months, separation anxiety is a normal part of infant development, but it can make a baby's introduction to substitute care difficult for all involved. If your baby gets anxious whenever you leave her sight, take extra care in helping her to become familiar and comfortable with your provider.

Reverse-Cycle Feeding

One behavioral change in babies that *is* due to having a mother who's away all day is a reversal of day and night sleeping and nursing patterns. By the age of eight to twelve weeks, a baby *may* have settled into a predictable pattern like this: Awake and alert all morning, she nurses two to four times between waking and midday, takes a long afternoon nap, and is awake in the late day and early evening. After dinner she sleeps for four or five hours, wakes and nurses once, and then sleeps for another three hours. But when her mother goes back to work, and the baby begins spending six to eight hours a day in substitute care, her pattern may change. She may sleep part of the morning and all afternoon at daycare. She may accept 8 ounces of expressed breast milk once in the middle of the day, but seems satisfied thereafter until her mother comes to pick her up. Then, *ta da!* She may be awake and alert all evening, wanting to socialize with her parents and nurse frequently. She may increase the number of times she wants to nurse from once or twice to three or four times a night. Her mother may wonder, "Why doesn't she ever nap at home anymore? Why isn't she sleeping through the night the way she used to?" and (of course) "What am I doing wrong?"

In studying working mothers and their babies, Irene Frederick and Kathleen Auerbach found that many well-attached babies sleep for longer periods during their mothers' absence and are wakeful when their mothers are present. These babies simply shift their schedules to nurse frequently when their mothers are available, and consequently may not need to be fed more than twice during an eight-hour separation. "You and your baby are a dyad," says Kittie Frantz, a pediatric nurse practitioner and lactation authority, "and are so well connected that the baby has adjusted as your body is adjusting." The baby simply goes into low gear while waiting for you. This is the highest compliment a nursing baby can give his mother; it is proof of a deep attachment between the two.

If your baby sleeps a lot and drinks little while you're at work, he will want to make up the missed daytime feedings with evening, nighttime, and early morning nursings. This can mean that, just after your baby has begun sleeping through most of the night, he resumes nursing several times a night again. Mothers whose babies sleep with them hardly notice the difference. The mother is getting all the rest she needs, her baby can nurse all he wants, and both mother's and baby's needs for physical contact with each other are fulfilled. If sharing a bed is not an option for you, nurse as long and as much as your baby would like in the early evening and morning, as well as once at night. Expect your baby to stay up much later than he might have before. If your baby feels physically and emotionally satiated during these hours he may keep his nursing to a minimum during the hours you would really like to have unbroken sleep.

A reversal of your baby's feeding cycle should mean less pumping for you. As one mother explained, "It seemed that all of my children would rather just tough it out until I came home from work; they wouldn't take anything from a bottle." If you pick up your baby at daycare to find, day after day, that he has not drunk all the milk you have left, you can adjust your pumping accordingly. You may even find that when your baby is five or six months old and has begun sampling solid foods, your stock of frozen milk will meet all your baby's daytime needs for breast milk, and you can reduce or even quit pumping altogether.

If your baby keeps with his old cycle, this doesn't mean that you are not deeply attached to each other. Your baby is probably one of those wonderfully flexible souls who adapts to new situations without batting an eye. But if reverse-cycle feeding sounds good to you, because it means less pumping, storing, and transporting milk, you can encourage your baby by putting him to the breast more often during the evening and just before you go to bed, even if he is asleep. Babies are quite able to nurse when in the "active" phase of sleep, which constitutes approximately half their sleeping hours. Your baby probably won't wake up fully to nurse, and will go right back to sleep afterward. If you wake up in the middle of the night while your baby is sleeping, have another brief, quiet nursing. Add one more to your morning routine. The more your baby nurses while you are together, the less milk you will need to leave with your daycare provider.

Pumping and Your Milk Supply

Pumping has a reputation for being an onerous burden, but once it becomes a part of your daily routine—and you are letting down your milk in response to its stimulation—it is hardly any trouble at all. Think of pumping as a respite and a time to focus on your baby no matter where you are or what else is going on.

Your milk supply is normally at its highest level in both volume and fat content in the early- and mid-morning and lowest in the late afternoon. Therefore, an early-morning pumping session, especially if your baby is still sleeping and you are quite full, will yield the most milk. A mid-morning pumping at work also will be productive, while your afternoon session may produce just half the midmorning amount.

If you fall into a pattern of nursing and pumping similar to the one in the example at the top of page 175, you will probably have at least 8 ounces of fresh milk for your baby each day. Remember, though, that *every mother-and-baby pair is different.* If your baby nurses more often than the baby in the example, or if you obtain a lot of milk during your morning pumping sessions, you may not need to pump in the afternoon at all. Your baby may soon sleep through the late-night nursing, too (if she has reversed her cycles, though, she may keep it up for quite a while).

If your baby is starting a growth spurt and requires more milk than you are pumping, you can supplement your fresh milk with frozen. If you pump more than your baby consumes in a day, add the extra to your frozen stocks. In the example, the mother's breasts are stimulated and drained seven to ten times in 24 hours, enough to

A TYPICAL DAY OF PUMPING AND NURSING FOR A MOTHER OF A FOUR-MONTH-OLD

5:00 A.M.	Nurse (and sleep).
6:00 A.M.	Pump both breasts. Yield: 2 to 4 ounces, to be saved for the following day or take to daycare that morning.
8:15 A.M.	Nurse briefly at daycare.
10:30 A.M.	Pump for 15 minutes at work. Yield: 4 to 7 ounces.
3:30 P.M.	Pump for 15 minutes at work. Yield: 2 to 5 ounces.
5:30 P.M.	Nurse at daycare.
6:00 P.M.	Nurse longer at home.
9:00 P.M.	Nurse.
1:00 A.M.	Nurse (and sleep).
5:00 A.M.	Nurse (and sleep).

maintain her milk production at the level she requires. In general, during the first four to five months after birth you will need to stimulate your breasts once every three to four hours while you and your baby are apart to prevent your milk supply from decreasing.

When your baby is four to six months old, and has grown as big as she is going to be without yet becoming interested in mashed bananas and applesauce, you are at your peak of milk production. Your baby will consume most of your milk at the breast, but your pumping is likely to be at a peak as well. During this period you will want to be sure to keep your own protein and fluid intake high—especially if you are simultaneously returning to work.

Your milk supply will vary over the course of a week. After nursing more frequently on the weekend, you may find yourself a little full on Monday morning. At the end of a workweek, you may find that your milk production seems a little low by Friday night. "Near the end of the week," recalls one mother, "my milk supply would go down. I nursed in bed a lot over the weekend so that I could rest and sleep while she built up my milk supply. On Mondays I had more milk and needed breast pads, but my supply was back to normal on Tuesdays." You may be able to counteract the fluctuations somewhat by decreasing your fluid intake on Sunday night and drinking more fluids all day Friday. But you'll find that your body is wonderfully sensitive to your baby's changing needs. As one mother says, "My body always seemed to know when it was the weekend." If you will not be pumping, extra nursing on weekends may be vital for rebuilding your supply for the coming week.

The nursing, working mother's rule: "My baby gets a bottle when I'm not there, and breastfeeds when I am there."

Your milk supply can be affected by catching a cold, missed meals, stress, and fatigue. Taking decongestants, some antihistamines, or estrogen-containing birth-control pills (or becoming pregnant, which also increases estrogen in your body) can diminish your milk production. Pumping, however, will help you keep your production up despite these things. If none of these seems to be a factor, yet your supply seems to be decreasing, consider the cycling rate of your pump (see Chapter 6, page 141). It may be cycling too slowly—not sucking as frequently as your baby does—and therefore not withdrawing the milk as efficiently. Try varying the speed of your pump, if possible, to match more closely your baby's sucking pattern over the course of a nursing session. One mother whose supply seemed to be decreasing recalls, "I realized that my daughter's sucking pattern had changed recently, so I tried mimicking her nursing pattern with the pump. When my flow slackened during a pumping session, I ran the pump on slow for a minute or two. Then I set it back up to medium, or fast and then medium. This gave me a second, but smaller, let-down." It is easy to adjust the cycling rate with an automatic pump; you can also do this with a manual pump, although you'll have to expend more effort. If you are unhappy with your pump in general, a different type or model may be the solution. See Chapter 6, pages 143–148, for suggestions.

Combining Breastfeeding and Formula Feeding

If you have decided to combine formula and nursing, and dispense with pumping, be certain to continue to nurse *at least* seven times, draining the breasts each time, every weekday until your baby is well-established on solid foods. Encourage long nursings, especially if it is hard to manage frequent ones. Nurse lying down so that you can rest and sleep while your baby is getting all the milk and skin-to-skin contact he needs. One way or the other, you will need at least two hours of nipple stimulation, let-down, and withdrawal per 24-hour period to maintain your supply, and three or more hours to increase it. Night nursing, and frequent nursing on the weekends, will help ensure that your milk production stays bountiful.

Combining formula feeding and nursing may be problematic, however, during a baby's periodic appetite spurts. Because formula takes longer to digest than breast milk, a sudden increase in appetite may not be apparent while the baby is at daycare. At home, though, the baby will want to nurse a great deal more than usual. If the baby's appetite seems satisfied at daycare and insatiable at home, you may assume that you can no longer produce enough milk to meet the baby's needs. And, because you are not pumping during the day, you'll take longer to build your supply. Even a temporarily inadequate milk supply can shake a mother's self-confidence. Understanding what is happening can help you weather such episodes, and frequent short nursing sessions on your days off will close the gap between your baby's increased appetite and your milk supply. But pumping during separations from your baby, if only for a day or two, is the best way to raise your milk production to meet your baby's increased appetite.

If you reduce the number of daily nursings, your milk supply may diminish to the point that the baby becomes frustrated at the breast. To keep him from rejecting the breast in favor of the bottle, you might have your caregiver feed him formula from a cup instead of a bottle.

If you are having a lot of trouble maintaining your milk supply, consider taking fenugreek capsules or fennel tea (see page 189).

Leaking

Your milk may have stopped dripping and spraying months ago but now that you are back at work you may be dealing with leaking milk all over again. Your breasts may leak when they are very full because you haven't been able to nurse or pump on your regular schedule, or even when something reminds you of your baby. (One mother found that her milk let down whenever she stepped into the elevator to go home to her baby. After a while her milk let down whenever she entered a descending elevator for any reason, forcing her to stand with crossed arms when she rode in one.) Once you establish a pumping schedule, your body will adjust, and leaking shouldn't be a problem any longer. Meanwhile, wear nursing pads in your bra to absorb any leaked milk (see Chapter 4, page 65).

You can stop a leak, when you feel your milk letting down, by gently pressing on your nipples until the let-down sensation subsides. Do this discreetly by crossing your arms and pushing the sides of your hands directly against your nipples and breasts to stop the milk flow. At your desk or a conference table, you can also put your elbows on the table in front of you and your hands under your chin and press the backs of your upper arms against your breasts.

As long as the leaking continues (which varies greatly from woman to woman), wear pads and clothes that will camouflage leaks. Printed fabrics are a good bet. You might also keep an extra jacket, sweater, vest, or long scarf at your workplace in case you need to throw it on to cover any spots.

Pumping at Work

The ease or difficulty of pumping at work depends on the nature of your workplace and your own comfort with your decision to nurse and pump. Regardless of how your coworkers feel about having someone pumping her breasts nearby, try to keep a relaxed attitude. Without being ashamed or secretive, you can keep your twice-a-day activity to yourself (since the newest pumps are so small and so quiet, and their cases discreet, this is easier than it once was). If someone asks about your pump or your brief disappearances, tell the truth. Pumping and storing milk at work may raise a few eyebrows, but not nearly so many as you might fear. One mother found that her colleagues reacted with fascination. "They wanted to see the milk, asked if it hurt to pump, and wanted to examine the pump," she said. If someone does voice disapproval, brush off the comments as you would any intrusion into your private life. You have chosen to do this for your baby and yourself; no one else's opinion matters. In all likelihood, your proud example will enlighten your colleagues and encourage other working mothers to breastfeed, too.

You may have no problem letting down your milk in response to the stimulation of your pump. Or you may find that, although your milk flows easily into the pump at home, pumping at work is less relaxing and less productive. Persevere; in time you will learn to relax and withdraw all the milk you need. Put a sign on the door of your pumping space that says, "Room available at 10:15" (or whenever you expect to be done). Unlike a "Do not disturb" sign or no sign at all, this tells the curious and the impatient all they need to know. Then you can erase thoughts of what is happening outside the room and turn your mind to your baby's lunch.

Set up a routine for pumping; it will calm your mind and help you to let down your milk. Begin just as you did at home when first learning to pump. Wash your hands and arrange your pump, pumping kit, and, perhaps, a picture of your baby in front of you. Keep a hand towel in your pump's carrying case to catch drips. For the first few days back at work you might bring along the shirt or sleeper your baby wore the night before, so you can breathe in his scent to stimulate your let-down. If it helps, you might imagine hearing your baby nursing, guzzling, murmuring, or even crying to be fed. You might hum lullabies, and lightly stroke your breasts with your fingertips. When you are relaxed and ready, fit the pump flange to your breast and turn on the pump. If you are using an automatic pump, begin with a fast cycle at low suction to mimic the way a baby begins nursing. Gradually increase suction while slowing down the cycle (although not below 48 cycles per minute). If you are using a manual pump, gently pump a few times until you feel your milk letting down, then hold the pump in its extended position and let your milk spray into it.

If you are using a single-side pump, switch your pump to the other breast when the spray slackens, and then back again. Switching back and forth will yield more milk than doing each side once. With a good let-down you may be able to collect as much as an ounce a minute. Strive to stimulate two let-downs per session.

Double-pumping—pumping both breasts at once—will probably yield more milk with less time and effort. One study found that double-pumping increases women's prolactin levels more than single-side pumping, causing more frequent and stronger let-downs and greater milk yield. Double-pumping also reduces the time required to pump from 15 to 20 minutes to 8 to 10 minutes.

After you are done pumping, store your milk in a refrigerator, freezer, or cooler. Rinse the pump parts that have been touched by milk with hot tap water, and put away the pump. Later, at home, you can wash the parts more thoroughly with hot, soapy water. Daily boiling of all washable pump parts is not necessary unless so stated by the manufacturer. The rubber gaskets soon become dry and cracked with repeated heating, thereby reducing the pump's suction.

As you keep up your pumping sessions, you will find that they become easier and easier, requiring less and less preparation and time and yielding more milk. Eventually pumping should take so little effort that you will be able to read or, with a one-handed pump, write or talk on the phone while pumping. At this point, your 15 minutes of pumping need not take you away from your work.

If you simply can't pump at work and you don't want to use formula, try pumping before your baby wakes in the morning and after her bedtime. You may be able to provide all the milk she needs in this way, or at least keep her formula feedings to a minimum. If your commute and schedule allow, see if you can visit your baby at lunchtime to nurse, or have your baby brought to you at work, and nurse in the middle of the day. A grade-school teacher whose husband worked at home and took care of their baby relied on this plan. Not only did her husband come by with the baby at noon every day so that she could nurse in the teacher's lounge, but he brought her a freshly packed lunch as well.

As your baby approaches his first birthday, you may be able to reduce the frequency of your pumping sessions without compromising your milk supply. At some time during the second half of your baby's first year, it may even be possible to eliminate pumping altogether. As long as you nurse frequently at home, and offer solids after nursing, you may continue to produce the milk your baby needs. (You can let your baby have formula, water, or juice along with solid food while at daycare. Note that cow's milk is not recommended until a baby is at least a year old.) Many working women breastfeed part time for as long as they and their babies desire, often right through toddlerhood, enjoying the closeness and intimacy of being part of a nursing couple despite the daily separations.

Transporting Your Milk

You do not need to freeze your milk as soon as you pump it, but you will want to chill it if more than four hours are going to pass before it is drunk or frozen, if your workplace is especially warm, if your commute is long and hot, or if leaving your milk out just makes you fret (see page 152 for guidelines on storing milk). You can put your milk in the freezer section of the company refrigerator, if there is one, so that it is half frozen by the time you leave work. If your drive is a short one, you won't need to insulate the milk in transit. Or skip freezing your milk altogether. Chill your bags of milk in the company refrigerator until the end of the day, then put them into a wide-mouth insulated bottle with crushed ice at the bottom for the ride to daycare. Or put your bags or bottles of pumped milk directly into the cooler compartment of your pump carrier, or into a separate small cooler or insulated lunch bag with a freezer pack.

Once you arrive at daycare, leave your (labeled) milk in the refrigerator to stay cool until your baby's lunch the next day.

Teaching Your Caregiver
about Breastfeeding

Your baby's caregiver will be handling your expressed breast milk even more than you will. Even if she breastfed her own children, she may have little or no experience with storing and thawing breast milk. If your caregiver is familiar only with formula-fed babies, you will need to explain that breast milk is digested much more completely and more quickly than formula. Exclusively breastfed babies, especially very young ones, may therefore want to eat smaller but more frequent meals than the formula-fed babies to whom she may be accustomed—although if your baby reverses his cycles he may take a bottle less often than the formula-fed babies. Daycare providers understandably need to organize their days, and scheduled feeding times are usually a part of that organization, but your baby is accustomed to being fed whenever he is hungry. Talk to your caregiver about this; be sure that she is willing to give your baby a bottle of expressed breast milk whenever he seems to want it.

Explain that one of the benefits of breastfeeding is that breastfed babies excrete less waste than formula-fed babies. Sometimes caregivers are surprised by the stools of breastfed babies. They are loose, yellowish or greenish, and mild, almost sweet, in odor—not at all like what one might find in the diaper of a formula-fed infant.

Also explain that breast milk looks different from, and thinner than, cow's milk or formula. Breast milk can look bluish when fresh, and tends to turn pale yellow (although the color can vary) when frozen. Explain that when it is left to sit, it will separate, and the cream will rise to the top. Explain that the caregiver should shake the bottle to mix in the cream before feeding the milk to your baby.

If the caregiver will be using frozen milk, ask her to thaw only as much as she thinks she will need at a time. Thawed milk is less stable than fresh and will spoil if left at room temperature all day. If the caregiver is going on an all-day outing with the children—to the playground, perhaps—she should take along a bottle of chilled fresh milk, which will keep much longer than thawed milk.

Show the caregiver how to thaw breast milk by letting the frozen bag sit in a cup of warm water for 15 minutes—and be sure she knows never to microwave breast milk. If you use milk storage bags or bottle liners, let her see how you open one, pour the milk into a feeding bottle, and shake the bottle to mix in the cream.

Ask your caregiver to help you to keep track of how much milk your baby is drinking so that you can pump accordingly. Tell her about "frequency days," when babies are extra hungry and would like to nurse all day; your caregiver may need to fit in an extra feeding at such times. Explain that she can draw on your frozen stores on those days—and that you'll value her judgment about how much more milk to provide.

Be sure that your caregiver understands that even on the hottest day of summer your exclusively breastfed baby does not need water in addition to breast milk. Your breast milk provides him with everything he needs until he is six months old. As your baby grows and begins to add solids to his diet, your caregiver should know that she can use breast milk, just as she might use formula for another baby, to mix with cereal or applesauce.

Finally, remind the caregiver that your baby may strenuously object to drinking on his own from a propped bottle. You are breastfeeding your baby for many reasons, one of which is the physical contact it provides. Breast or bottle, he still needs to be held and cuddled at mealtimes. Consistency in care will help your baby adjust to your separations with a minimum of stress.

Your caregiver will want detailed instructions on how to thaw and warm breast milk, and what to do with milk left in the bottle (see Using Stored Milk, page 156). Write these instructions out so that she can put them up on the wall and refer to them easily.

Caregivers sometimes have a tendency to overfeed babies while their mothers are at work, perhaps giving the babies as much milk during an 8- to 10-hour period as they would normally take over an entire day. When a baby is fussy, everyone's first impulse is to feed him, although the baby may not actually be hungry or thirsty. Teach your caregiver to spot the cues that your baby gives when he is hungry, rather than sleepy or frazzled. Does he root to the side with his mouth or gnaw on his fist? The more sensitive your caregiver is to his early signals of hunger, the less she'll need to soothe his crying and the more easily she'll be able to tell when he is truly hungry or not. Include in your written instructions a note about how much milk you expect your baby will want during the day, and how often. Most breastfed babies need milk about every two to three hours. If they are hungry every two hours, they'll probably take about three ounces of milk in a feeding. If it's been three hours since the last feeding, they may take four and a half ounces. As babies grow, of course, they take more at each feeding. You want to avoid, however, a situation developing in which most of your baby's calories are coming from bottles of expressed milk at daycare, rather than directly from the breast at home. It's okay to ask your caregiver to try to settle your baby with walking, rocking, or a pacifier, if he's already taken several ounces of milk and still seems unhappy.

If your caregiver would like to give your baby an especially filling, high-calorie meal, perhaps at noon before your baby takes a long nap, she can do so by making a double-cream feeding from your supply of expressed milk. When you store your milk in a transparent container, you will see where the cream has risen to the top. After thawing milk from two containers, pour off the cream from both, and combine them in a third container, leaving the thinner foremilk, the skim milk, for another feeding. The extra-rich feeding may keep your baby satiated for a good part of the time while you are at work, or can help tide her through a growth spurt while your milk supply is catching up.

Talk, too, to your caregiver about how you will manage at pick-up time. It is a poor end to a working mother's day when she arrives at daycare full of milk, desperate to nurse and hold her baby, and discovers he's just been fed. You want your baby ready to nurse as soon as he is back in your arms, before leaving daycare if possible, and again as soon as you are home. Ask your caregiver not to feed him in the last hour before pick-up time. If she absolutely must feed him because he's woken up early from his nap and is famished, she can give him the skim portion of stored milk, with the cream poured off (and saved!). The skim milk will satisfy him for a time, but he should still have enough appetite to nurse when you arrive. Confirm with your caregiver that it is not a problem if you sit with your baby quietly to nurse for 15 minutes or so before heading home.

Preventing and Treating
Plugged Ducts and Mastitis

Plugged ducts and breast infections plague some mothers. An employed mother is most likely to experience them during her first month or two back at work. Her milk is suddenly not being withdrawn as consistently or as well as it was during her maternity leave. She may be stressed and fatigued, increasing her risk of infection.

In one survey of nursing mothers, one-third reported that a period of fatigue and stress had preceded their mastitis. The rule for the mother of the newborn also applies to the mother recovering from a plugged duct or breast infection: if you're standing, then sit; sitting, then lie down; lying down, then sleep. And be sure that you are getting all the nutritious food and vitamins you need. For further advice on preventing and treating plugged ducts and mastitis, see pages 68-72.

HOW TO TREAT PLUGGED DUCTS OR A BREAST INFECTION

◆ Take off your bra, and go to bed.

◆ Nurse as much as the baby is willing, starting on the affected breast. Position the baby with her chin pointing at the sore spot.

◆ Apply moist warm compresses, and massage your breasts toward the nipple.

◆ Drink plenty of fluids.

◆ If you have a fever lasting 12 hours or more, call your doctor. You may need antibiotics.

Adjusting to Being Away from Your Baby

Missing your baby will probably be the hardest part of going back to work. Your first full day without your baby may be truly wrenching. But you can draw comfort from your breastfeeding relationship, which is proof that you and your baby are indispensable to each other. Each pumping session at work will remind you of this. Remember, too, that intensely missing your baby is a sign that you are well attached, and that therefore your work cannot distance you emotionally from your baby.

Just as your baby needs to be both physically and emotionally satiated by breastfeeding and contact with you, you need your full dose of your baby each day. As long as you are not working extraordinarily long hours, you make up for the missed hours at home by nursing, carrying your baby in a sling or baby pack, and socializing with her. Letting your baby sleep with you can dramatically increase the close contact between the two of you, making the hours that you are apart much easier to bear. When you're at home, concentrate on understanding and answering your baby's needs rather than fostering her "independence." Staying in harmony with your baby will make the separations less difficult, and your work may soon become a comfortable part of your routine.

As your baby grows and develops over the amazing first year of her life, so will you continue to grow and develop as her mother. Stay sensitive to the changes within you. Find ways to integrate the lessons you are learning as a mother into the other parts of your life, and wear your motherhood with pride. After spending several years helping to launch an exciting new publishing company, a distinguished editor and writer decided to return to her independent work. Addressing the staff at her goodbye party, she declared that being a part of the launch had been "one of the grandest adventures of my life, one matched only by being a mother." Appreciate your own grand adventure through motherhood, and garner the rich awards it can give you.

The lessons of breastfeeding in particular can linger long beyond weaning. Most important, breastfeeding teaches the subtle but valuable lesson of receptivity. As Karen Pryor writes in *Nursing Your Baby*, "Think of the difference between 'passive' and 'receptive.' There is partnership implicit in being receptive that is the very nature of the nursing relationship." Approaching your family members and the people with whom you work with the receptivity you have learned through breastfeeding, as a *partner* open to their cues, will enrich your relationships. Trusting yourself as you have trusted that your body can nourish your baby will make every new challenge less daunting. The intuition that guides you in caring for your baby will thus serve you well in all areas of your life, if you let it.

Making Enough Milk

Every mother frets at some point about whether she is producing enough milk for her baby. At five to six months, breastfed babies are taking more milk than before or than they will after they add solids to their diet. This peak in their appetites coincides with the first couple of months back at work for many mothers. A worried working mom may assume that a baby is ravenous not because he is growing by leaps and bounds, but because she isn't supplying enough milk. If your pump is efficient and you are producing 8 to 12 ounces a day with it, you are probably making more than enough milk for your baby's needs at daycare. Most lactating women will produce, on average, about 1½ ounces per hour over the course of 24 hours.

If you are concerned, however, that your supply isn't keeping up with your baby's consumption at daycare, consider first the possibility that your caregiver is overfeeding him (see pages 184–85). If your baby takes more than 1½ ounces per hour, some adjustments may need to be made. Nurse your baby, if possible, at daycare when you first take him there to top off his breakfast, and plan to nurse him again as soon as you are reunited. Prepare bottles of expressed milk with specified amounts for single feedings to help your caregiver give an appropriate amount at each meal. You can also try switching to a slower-flow nipple so that your baby's meals last a little longer and are more satisfying. If general fussiness is leading your caregiver to overfeed your baby, try to identify the reasons for his crankiness, and suggest other tried and true ways to soothe your baby. Perhaps your baby just needs to be carried more. Giving your caregiver a sling or frontpack in which to carry him while she attends to other children may meet both their needs. If your baby is six months old, or close to it, she also can begin offering him solids to supplement your expressed breast milk.

If you really are producing insufficient milk, or your milk supply seems to be decreasing, you can solve this problem, too. Be sure that, between nursing and pumping, you are draining both your breasts at least seven times a day. The most efficient way to increase milk production is to nurse as often as possible when you and your baby are together, especially at night when your prolactin levels are highest. If your baby is sleeping most of the night, you may wish to nurse him at 11:00 P.M. or 12:00 A.M., without fully wakening him, just to get an extra session in.

If your supply is dropping after a few weeks back at work, take a close look at your breast pump. Does it fully drain your breasts? Are you using a high-quality, fully automatic pump that cycles between 48 and 60 times a minute (see pages 141–42)? Are the flanges on your accessories kit, the funnels that press against your breasts, large enough for your breasts and areola? You can check this by pumping as usual and then, 20 to 30 minutes later, pumping a second time. If you pump more than a half ounce in the second session, your pump may not be draining your breasts as it should.

Many mothers have found that taking fenugreek helps counter low milk production. A spice used in Indian cuisine, fenugreek is known to stimulate milk production. It is well tolerated by nursing mothers and babies, and it has only one side effect: It causes a mother's sweat and urine to take on the distinct scent of maple syrup. Available at health-food stores, fenugreek capsules are usually taken three at a time, three times a day. Most mothers notice a boost in milk production in about 48 hours. A few other spices, such as fennel, are thought to be helpful in increasing milk production. The Motherlove Herbal Company (see Resources, page 217) offers tinctures as well as capsules of fenugreek combined with other lactation-stimulating spices.

Estrogen can decrease a mother's milk supply. Are you taking a low-dose estrogen-based birth control pill? If so, talk to your doctor about switching to the mini-pill or a progestin-only pill, which will not affect your milk production. Pregnancy can also decrease your milk supply, and your production may dip just before your period starts. Some lactation consultants suggest that a calcium-magnesium supplement, taken daily from mid-cycle through the end of your period, can help prevent this effect.

Business Travel

If your job requires you to travel at some point during the first year after your baby's birth, you do not need to wean your baby. If your trip comes before your baby is five or six months old, the easy solution is to take him along. Will you be in meetings all day? The hotel you stay at may be able to help you find a sitter. Do you have friends or family in the area to which you're traveling who can care for your baby while you work? Or can your husband, mother, or friend come with you? If your trip is to a large city or resort area, he or she and the baby can take in the sights while you work. Meetings at most conferences last two or three hours, with just enough time in between to run up to your room, or meet your husband, mother, or sitter somewhere, and nurse the baby. Bringing someone along to help you with the baby will add substantially to the cost of your trip, but will make it considerably easier. If bringing the baby along would scandalize your employer, just don't publicize the fact that you're doing it. The presence of your baby in your hotel room is not going to affect your performance in the conference room or the exhibit hall.

You might even wear your baby while you work. If you can do this with confidence, meeting your baby's needs without interrupting other activities, your only barrier may be the necessity of keeping up a "professional image." Perhaps you will be among the growing number of women who are inventing a new professionalism that incorporates the presence of contented babies and cooperative children.

Unfortunately, many business trips require 12- to 15-hour days of intense concentration and hard work. If you are meeting new clients, making sales pitches, or visiting laboratories or factories, bringing your baby along probably isn't an option, no matter how confident you are. The ease of traveling without your baby depends on how old he is and how much milk your body is making. If you cannot take your baby, make your trip as short as possible for both your sakes. If he is younger than six months, he is probably still nursing seven or more times a day and will require a stored milk supply of at least 32 ounces per day. You may wish to supplement with formula, if your baby will drink it, so that your frozen stocks are not used up all at once. However, providing for a two-day separation could be the best use of your stored supply.

You will need to pump your milk nearly as often as your baby nurses to avoid becoming uncomfortably engorged with milk. You might be surprised to learn how much milk you are making, and how engorged you can become, when your baby is not there to remove it. Pack an effective portable pump, and find a way to take pumping breaks once in the early morning, twice during the day, and at least twice at night. Arrange your schedule to allow for these breaks, just as you would schedule in any other appointment. Pumping on a long plane ride may be the stiffest challenge of the trip. Airplane bathrooms barely have enough room to accomplish the purpose for which they are intended, much less for setting up a pump and expressing milk. Ask your partner or a friend to see you off, and nurse your baby in the airport if possible. If your flight is five hours or less, you probably can wait until you reach your destination before pumping. If you have a very long flight in front of you, bring along a hand pump. You may wish to practice with it beforehand, since hand pumps can be frustrating to use if you haven't learned how. A hand pump is a good choice for small spaces, since these pumps need not be set on a table to operate, can be tucked into a purse, and can be rinsed out with hot water in a small sink.

You may wish to discard your expressed milk (as wrenching as this can be) to simplify matters, rather than worrying about adequate refrigeration while you are on the move. If you want to save the milk you pump, you may wish to bring along a small picnic cooler, or invest in one of the coolers made especially for expressed breast milk, so that you can transport a large quantity of milk easily. Please note that airline regulations may prevent you from carrying fluids, even breast milk, on board unless your baby is traveling with you. Consider instead packing your milk in blue ice and sending it home by overnight delivery each day.

When your baby is older than six months, traveling becomes somewhat easier. Your baby may be supplementing his breastfeeding with solids and nursing less or not at all at night. You may still need to pump three or four times a day while you're away but you are less likely to become engorged and uncomfortable.

Your milk production probably will decrease over the course of even a two- or three-day trip if your pump is inefficient or if you've pumped infrequently. Take a couple of days off work afterward, if at all possible, to be with your baby, nurse frequently, and build back up your supply.

Deciding When to Stop Expressing

When will you put away the pump for good? Depending on your baby's growth rate and diet of solids, the steadiness of your milk supply, and the demands of your schedule, you may wish to stop pumping (but keep nursing) some time in the second half of your baby's first year. Babies should have either their mother's milk or formula through their first birthday, so you may wish to continue pumping and producing your baby's breast milk lunch until then. Or your baby may have lunches of infant cereal, applesauce, and sips of water when at daycare. If you are separated from your baby for no more than six to eight hours a day, stopping pumping may be possible.

Mothers often continue expressing their milk for continued immunological protection while their babies are in daycare. Daycare exposes babies to viruses and other infections, and breast milk protects against these even after six months. If you are approaching cold and flu season, you may wish to put off your break with the pump until the season is past.

When you decide to stop expressing milk, you will want to do so slowly, especially if you have a well-established milk supply and you are away from your baby for more than 20 hours each week. An abrupt stop could make you uncomfortably engorged, and engorgement could lead to plugged milk ducts and mastitis. Eliminate your afternoon pumping session for a couple of weeks. When you feel your breasts have adjusted to the decreased demand, pump in the morning as usual, but for half the time. Then, in a few days, stop pumping altogether.

Weaning

In most traditional societies, children are usually completely weaned somewhere between eighteen months and four years of age, but never before the end of the first year. American babies are rarely nursed beyond six months, despite the American Academy of Pediatrics' recommendation that all babies be nursed for a full year and beyond as long as both mother and baby desire. Babies are weaned early in our society for many reasons, some of which are simply justifications for the fact that people are uncomfortable seeing an older baby or toddler still nursing. Working mothers do tend to wean earlier than other mothers because they receive less support for nursing and more pressure to divide their lives into incompatible spheres. Your baby need not wean any earlier than he might if you were not working.

If your milk supply was well established before you returned to work and began pumping, you should be able to produce as much milk as your baby wants indefinitely. Allow your baby to continue to nurse for comfort as well as for food, and breastfeeding will be a way for you and your child to reconnect after your separations for as long as you both wish. Nursing into the second year or longer offers significant emotional benefits to children as they begin to experience life's bumps and bruises.

When you do wish to wean, keep in mind that weaning is a significant developmental milestone, like crawling, walking, or eating solids, and that it rarely happens all at once. Sometimes parents treat weaning as if it were like quitting smoking. They try to follow a regimen that subtracts one nursing each week until the baby isn't nursing at all. But infants don't develop on a rigid schedule, and breastfeeding isn't an addiction. Watch how your baby progresses through other developmental stages. Milestones are almost always reached gradually, with two steps forward, then one step back. This is why parents often recognize their children's developmental progress only in retrospect.

Very occasionally a baby gives up nursing over the course of just a few days. Perhaps a new tooth or an earache has made her reluctant to nurse (or to eat anything); somehow, when she is feeling better, she and her mother have moved on to a stage of life that does not include nursing. Or a baby may come to prefer the bottle because her mother's milk supply is low, although she would prefer nursing if she could get a good meal out of it. Or a baby might suddenly refuse to nurse because of something in her mother's diet that is making the milk taste odd or is causing an allergic reaction, or because of thrush or another infection. In all these cases, weaning may not be the baby's intention, but it happens anyway. Often her mother has seized the opportunity to wean her baby quickly.

Ideally, a nursing relationship evolves gradually over the course of six months or more into one that is just as close but in which breastfeeding is no longer a part. When this happens, neither mother nor baby may remember when they nursed for the last time. The mother may realize that her baby, whether one year, one and a half, or two and a half years old, hasn't nursed for three or four days. Perhaps he will want to nurse again in a week or so when he stubs his toe. She might let him, or she might distract him with a hug and a cookie. In another week or month, she realizes that he is truly weaned. In most cases of gradual weaning, a mother uses gentle encouragement and creative substitutes for nursings as the baby becomes interested in other things.

Mothers as well as babies benefit from gradual weaning. Sudden weaning may bring with it an emotional letdown, by ending all at once the production of the nursing hormones and their soothing effects. Sudden weaning may even lead to serious depression, perhaps when the abrupt end of lactation causes an overload of minerals in the bloodstream. Gradual weaning helps avoid these effects.

Weaning also requires adjusting to the loss of the rest times that come with nursing—the excuse to lie down with the baby and relax. If your baby is very active, you may miss the physical intimacy of nursing, especially as your baby becomes a busy toddler with little time for cuddling. And, since weaning means losing your automatic cry-stopper, you will have to find other ways to comfort your baby as he grows. All of these changes are easier to adjust to when they are gradual. Over time, you can replace nursing breaks with quiet times spent napping or looking at books together.

If you wish that your baby would hurry things up a bit, however, you are not alone. No matter how much a woman has enjoyed breast-feeding, a time comes when she is ready to move on to the next stage of mothering. If you feel ready to be done with nursing, you can encourage gradual weaning.

If you are weaning a child one year old or older, choose a nursing that seems to matter less to your baby than others during the day, and casually substitute a cup of milk or juice (a choice between chocolate milk and a nursing can work wonders with toddlers).

Postponing a nursing works well for some toddlers. Ask your child to wait for his morning nursing until you get to the daycare provider's house, where he may be swept up in the day's activities and forget all about nursing.

With these gentle distractions, you can reduce nursing to the one session per day that really matters to your child, probably the bedtime or early-morning nursing. This last nursing may linger for several months. At bedtime your husband may be able to help by putting your baby to bed for a couple of weeks, until he has forgotten about his end-of-the-day nursing. If the baby screams for you, Dad might try taking him for a walk or drive at bedtime in hopes that he will fall asleep on the way.

The Nursing Mother's Guide to Weaning by Kathleen Huggins and Linda Ziedrich has numerous suggestions for coaxing your baby to wean when you are ready.

Falling Apart

Sometimes, between six months and a year after her baby is born, a working mother may feel herself falling to pieces. Although in the eyes of everyone else she has managed beautifully, she feels as if she cannot manage another second. After all, she is working or on call 24 hours a day. All her activities and most of her thoughts are dedicated to meeting other people's needs. Her day is scheduled to the last minute. She hasn't found more than 20 minutes to herself in the last week, and when she says so people assume she is exaggerating. One evening she may find herself in tears, confessing to her partner or a friend on the phone that she "can't do it anymore. I cannot meet another need. I cannot take on one more responsibility."

In addition, just when she has got used to caring for a newborn whose needs—"feed me, change me, hold me, love me"—may have been constant but were relatively simple, she now has an older baby with a mind of his own, and the increasing mobility to satisfy it. Now Mom's on her feet as the baby explores everything he can reach with grasping hands and open mouth. She thought she had completed the adjustment to motherhood, but at six months she realizes that there is yet another stage to traverse—and yet more after this one stretch into the distance.

The realities of motherhood have sunk in with a thunk. Yes, your life has changed irrevocably. It will get easier someday in the future. For the time being, however, acceptance, rather than resistance, will help you to cope. Now that you are a mother, you can't flop down on the sofa with a magazine when you get home from work anymore. You can't be sure that your plans won't be thrown into the air like a deck of cards at the last minute because your baby has a fever or because the daycare provider unexpectedly closes her doors for the day. You aren't in total control of your life—and you won't have as much control as you'd like until your children are grown.

Although at-home mothers can also fall apart six months to a year after their babies are born, working mothers tend to find this time especially challenging. If you have been used to being in control at work, now, like all parents, you are facing the fact that babies and children aren't controllable; they're their own persons. Lack of control is frustrating and worrisome. We tend to respond to it by seeking more control.

In parenting, however, control isn't always the answer. You may find that you can ride out crises and other unpredictable events with flexibility and a sense of humor. This takes practice and an open mind, but the ability to say, "Ah, well—let's move on to plan B (or D, or Z)," or even, "Let's make it up as we go along," will serve you well at home and at work. Breastfeeding teaches this lesson well. (While learning to nurse, how many times did you think, "Well, if this position isn't working today, let's try another," or "Gee, I thought you were full; but if you would like to nurse again, that's fine"?)

Lack of time for yourself goes hand in hand with feeling out of control. It would be easier to be flexible if you could just get a break once in a while. Find ways to increase your efficiency and simplify your life at home (see Managing Life at Home, page 198) so you'll have more time to do what you like. The working mother may actually have more opportunities for building in time for herself than many at-home mothers. She has a daily lunch break, as much as an hour (what riches!) to do whatever she wants. Many working mothers confess that one of the joys of coming to work is being able to go to the bathroom whenever they want, *alone* and with the door *closed.*

If the six-month crisis hits you, find other mothers with whom you can talk. They know that you aren't exaggerating when you say you had only 20 minutes to yourself last week. With support from your friends, that end-of-your-rope feeling may be a brief though intense phase in your adjustment to motherhood.

Or your distress may compel you to re-evaluate the decisions you have made about working. Perhaps you don't want to work full time after all. Reread pages 128–31 for ideas on redesigning your job to better fit into your life. More and more people are doing this; maybe you can, too. Whether a passing phase or a true crisis, feeling like you're falling apart is always a signal that you need to take care of yourself before you can take care of anyone else.

Managing Life at Home

"How," you may ask, "can I add taking care of myself to my list of responsibilities when I am already overwhelmed?" Savvy moms have found ways. At home, search out ways of taking five- to ten-minute breaks. Deborah Shaw Lewis, author of *Motherhood Stress,* writes that these mini-vacations are "golden moments, and they are almost always unexpected. You may not be able to plan them, so you have to watch for them. Suddenly you realize the baby is asleep, the kids are all playing a game, or there is absolute silence in the house. Take advantage of that. Consciously relax your body and say to yourself, 'Hey, I'm on vacation.'"

Try not to let your favorite pastime—gardening, playing music, hiking—languish during this busy first year. You can still do many such activities whether your baby decides to take a nap or not. Just put her in a sling or a baby pack and carry on. One mother plays her piano every evening while her six-month-old sits in a backpack looking over her shoulder, spellbound by her mother's dancing fingers and the wonderful sounds they make.

To save time, look for opportunities to do two or more things at once. Clean the kitchen or fold laundry while talking on the phone (cordless phones are a big help). While waiting at the post office, the gas station, the pharmacy, or in the grocery line, make a to-do list or a shopping list, balance your checkbook, write a postcard, or update your calendar. Do some stretching while your baby and any older children play in the park. While wearing your baby in a sling or baby pack, cook dinner, talk on the phone, fold laundry, or pick things up around the house. If you use a computer, you may be able to get a lot of work done while wearing your baby. Your baby may be just as fascinated by your fingers on a keyboard and the flickering dots and lights of your computer screen as the baby of that pianist is fascinated by her playing.

As satisfying as it is to find ways to increase your productivity, you must also allow yourself to *decrease* productivity. Worrying about all the things you should do will wear you down. If a bed is left unmade or an errand not run, forget about it. The bed is going to be slept in again very soon, anyway. You can probably run the errand later in the week. Notice how often you tell yourself, "I should be doing this or that," and stop yourself from thinking it. You are not doing "this or that" now, and if it becomes a real priority then you *will* do it . . . maybe.

Simplify. List your activities and responsibilities for an average week. Which ones can you eliminate, share with someone else, or move to a more convenient time? Screen calls with your answering machine. Have your phone number added to the National Do Not Call Registry, to keep telemarketers at bay. Keep a chalkboard or hanging pad of paper in a regular place so that you, your partner, and any older children can jot down household supplies that are running low. Check the list before you run errands or go grocery shopping. Use a grocery delivery service, if there is one in your area; the delivery fee is usually nominal. Invest in a large freezer to store precooked meals or prepared foods.

Appreciate the amount of work you do. How many of the following jobs are you primarily responsible for in your household? Cleaning the house, picking up daily clutter, bathing the baby, washing the dishes, arranging for babysitters, making doctor's appointments, driving children to school and daycare, cooking meals and packing lunches, buying clothes for the family, remembering relatives' birthdays and sending gifts, feeding and training pets, gardening, watering houseplants, doing the laundry and taking clothes to the dry cleaner, grocery shopping, keeping medical and financial records, keeping tabs on supplies that are running low, paying bills, buying stamps, planning menus, organizing play dates, opening and responding to mail, staying in touch with adult friends, and making social plans for you and your partner. Most or all of them, right? And you probably can add a few other duties to this already breathtaking list.

The problem with the work of motherhood is that so much of it is invisible, especially when it is done well. Besides your happy and healthy children, there is no product to show for your efforts, and very little recognition for them. And yet mothering is hard, constant work. Write a list of the jobs you do—the baby care, the household chores, and the paid work—and read it whenever you feel you aren't getting anything done. It will remind you how much you really do accomplish. Consider posting the list on the refrigerator so that others, especially your partner, will see all that you put into keeping the house and caring for the family. How many of these responsibilities can he take over?

Finally, learn to live in the moment. The years when your children are little pass quickly, but leave deep imprints on both you and your children. Savor these days while you are living them. All too soon your babies will be grown.

> " It is good to have an end to the journey; but it is the journey that matters in the end. "
>
> —URSULA LE GUIN

Managing at Work

Becoming a mother may make you ruthlessly efficient at work. After all, you cannot hang around the office until seven or eight o'clock putting the finishing touches on a project or chatting with colleagues. The efficiency you are learning at home will spill over into your paid work and help you finish tasks in less time. Office chitchat becomes less of a distraction and instead a rare indulgence.

The daily schedule of a working mother can be tyrannical. If you are not out the door and on your way to the babysitter's by 7:45, you will be late for work (again). You have exactly 15 minutes to travel from work to daycare or else you will be late to pick up your child (again). Many mothers find that their chief source of stress is all the times when the corners don't quite meet—when, for example, they have only 5 minutes instead of 15 to make it to daycare. Those 5 minutes, if they turn into 20 minutes in traffic, alone can deliver a full day's worth of strain and pressure. Other people can intensify such pressure. If you've left a late-running meeting early to arrive at daycare 10 minutes late, you may endure negative reactions on both ends.

Try to estimate realistic time requirements for every stage and transition in your day, and then pad your estimates. Other people may want you to be where they wish when they wish, but *you need to command your own schedule as much as possible in order to minimize each day's stress.* If at all possible, arranging a flextime schedule at work is an ideal way to achieve this autonomy. Don't apologize for leaving while others are staying late; just explain that you must be at daycare on time. Hiding the facts of your motherhood isn't good for you, your baby, or your coworkers. Work out a flexible arrangement with your daycare provider so that being 5 to 10 minutes late *once in a while* will not upset her. Offer to pay for these extra minutes, even if you don't end up using them. You need to focus on your baby during your departures and arrivals at daycare, not on conflicts between you and your provider.

Although you may be more efficient and doing better work than ever, you may find that you are still being taken less seriously at work than you once were. Perhaps this is because you leave at five o'clock sharp or because you have begun working on a flexible or part-time schedule. Your pumping breaks may leave more of an impression on the minds of your coworkers than someone else's slipping out to smoke a cigarette. Perhaps people automatically doubt your commitment to your job because you are now a mother.

You can counteract any perceptions that you may not be working as hard as you once did, without submitting to the urge to camouflage your motherhood. Write a memo summarizing each project you complete, and put a copy on the desk of anyone even vaguely connected to the project. When something comes up at home that requires a change of plans at work, offer several solutions at the time you present the problem. If your baby is running a fever and must stay home from daycare, call in during the day to discuss ongoing projects at work. If you know that you are going to be out for a few days, leave a stack of completed work in your out-box, and arrange for someone to cover your responsibilities while you are gone.

When you feel discouraged by the challenges of combining work and mothering, think about all that you are learning and gaining during this vigorous time of your life. Appreciate the ways that working is good for you and your family. First, it brings in essential income. It also offers the satisfaction of completing projects (and receiving monetary rewards and public recognition for doing so), something that motherhood rarely offers. In addition, working enables you to socialize with other adults every day. Conversations with colleagues can be relaxing and fun, and are something at-home mothers miss a great deal.

Consider also the ways in which the work you do as a parent enhances the work you do for pay. Every businessperson could benefit from the lessons of motherhood. As Katherine Ellison writes in *The Mommy Brain: How Motherhood Makes Us Smarter*, "What subsets of skills that can lend value to most professions might a practiced mother claim? I suggest four stand out: an ability to coordinate a variety of tasks under pressure, dependability, leadership, and caregiving." Ellison cites a 2003 Wellesley College report on senior female executives that reveals 20 percent credited their lives as mothers as a "training ground for leadership." Forty percent spoke of the leadership style of their most respected colleagues as similar to mothering. Every seasoned mother knows how to use her time efficiently, to set priorities, to delegate authority, to listen, to motivate others, to cooperate, to be dependable, to handle crises calmly, and above all to be patient and positive. Every experienced mother can do six or more things at once—and do them well. Anybody who has quizzed a child preparing for a spelling test, wiped down the kitchen counters and loaded the dishwasher, refereed a sibling squabble, answered the phone, mentally run through the errands to be done the next day, made a grocery list, kissed a toddler's stubbed toe (and found the preferred cartoon-character bandage to put on it), and noticed that the dog needs water—all within the same 15 minutes—is well prepared for a high-pressure job. Dive into this demanding period of your life. You will emerge stronger and more able than you ever thought possible.

When Your Baby Is Sick

Waking up on a weekday morning to find that a child is running a fever or throwing up and cannot go to daycare is a dreaded event for working parents. The solutions vary. Sometimes couples will "split the day" when a child is suddenly sick, one heading off to work as early as possible and coming home at noon so that the other can leave and stay as late as he or she needs to. If your work allows you to function by e-mail and telephone, you may be able to accomplish being in two places at once. Your allotted sick days, if you have a limited number, should apply to days when your children are not feeling well as much as when you're not well.

Your backup caregiver may or may not be able to step in. A day at Grandma's house is another solution, but Grandma may be heading out the door to her own job, or may live on the other side of the country. When a child is sick he usually and very much wants a parent with him. A breastfed baby feeling under the weather may be consoled by nothing but nursing. A sick older baby may even give up solids for a few days and temporarily obtain all his calories from breast milk.

When your child is suddenly sick, try to keep your perspective. Yield to the situation. Take the day off to hold and nurse your baby. If he is fighting an infection, he will need the extra nursing and cuddling to get better as quickly as possible.

> 66 Setting my priorities and being true to myself has given me peace of mind, if not always happiness. Apologize to no one; it's your life. 99
>
> —A MOTHER

Under any circumstances, don't dose your baby with Tylenol and send her to daycare because "she is just going to sleep most of the day, anyway." Your baby may have caught the bug from another child at daycare, but your provider needs all the help she can get in controlling the passing of germs among the children for whom she cares. Parents who knowingly bring sick children to daycare are the bane of daycare providers.

If your child needs you at home for an extended period, and his need puts your job at risk, you may be able to take advantage of the federal Family Medical Leave Act, which requires employers with 50 employees or more to allow 12 unpaid weeks off for any employee who needs to care for a dependent. (You may not be entitled to this leave, however, if your request falls in the same calendar year as your maternity leave did.) Smaller companies are not required to comply with the act, but if yours is very dependent on you it may be willing to work out a temporary leave, flextime schedule, or work-at-home arrangement until the crisis passes.

Bringing Your Baby to Work

What about bringing your baby to work with you, when daycare isn't available? If you work in a factory, hospital, laboratory, store, or restaurant, this may not be possible. But if you work in an office or other safe, private environment, bringing your baby along with you may be an option if she has a fairly innocuous but contagious illness like conjunctivitis or if she is well but her caregiver must take a day off. At a minimum, you might want to come in with the baby to pick up work to bring home and do while your baby naps.

You may also be able to get quite a lot of work done right in the office with your baby with you. If she is not very sick, just being near you may keep her happy most of the time. As at home, you can wear your baby in a sling, frontpack, or backpack while you do your desk or computer work. Or bring along a bouncy seat and a few interesting toys, and let her play at your feet as you work. Because you have encouraged a secure attachment since her birth, your baby is far more likely to play independently as long as you are near than would a baby who never gets enough of her mother.

Self-employed women or telecommuters with home offices are usually masters at blending work and mothering. Their experience offers practical ideas for every working parent. "As soon as my husband leaves, my baby and I 'get to work,'" says a freelance graphic designer. "If she's awake I put her on a baby blanket or in the frontpack, and use that time to talk on the phone to clients or suppliers. As soon as she naps, I go to my drafting table and do the work that requires creativity and intense concentration. I know that I can do certain kinds of work with my baby awake and other kinds only when she is asleep or with my husband. So I work around her schedule and am prepared to rearrange my plans whenever necessary."

A public relations specialist also arranges her work to harmonize with the rhythm of her baby's day. "I structure my time like this: Mornings when she is up and busy, I do lots of work on the cordless phone. After lunch it's naptime, and I sit at the computer and do work that requires concentration." An editor wakes up at 4:00 A.M. and does her most demanding work until the baby wakes at 6:00 A.M. Whatever happens the rest of the day, the most challenging portion of her work was completed before breakfast.

Breastfeeding streamlines baby care while you're working. A city planner advises, "As far as incorporating an eight-month-old into your work, I would suggest that this is much easier if you are breast-feeding. When my little one was tired of amusing herself, I could nurse her and continue to do whatever I was working on. I'm a great one-handed typist as a result!" She adds, "Now that my daughter is a toddler, I still bring her everywhere and hold her and cuddle her whenever possible. She's learned to join in if she can or to sit snugly on my lap, or in the sling when I'm occupied with work. It's the physical closeness that she really needs."

If your baby identifies your work as an opportunity to be close to you rather than an activity that takes you away from him, he is more likely to grow into a child who is happy to be near you while you work without demanding your undivided attention.

Blending Working and Mothering

"The key to combining working and mothering," says a freelance journalist, "is not to set yourself up for failure—for anger at your child or yourself, for feelings of frustration and anxiety and guilt. Keep a list of what you've gotten accomplished, but not a list of ideal goals. The ebb and flow is more productive than you think." This is the secret—knowing that working with an "ebb and flow" rhythm is just as productive, and often more so, than dedicating definite chunks of time to particular tasks. They are both valid, fruitful methods of working. Whether you can work productively while caring for your children depends on your attitude toward your work as much as how you keep your children busy and happy. Be flexible about when and how and where you work, and you may find that in the end you get as much done as if you had employed a rigid schedule and method.

A consultant to a nonprofit organization points out that being a part of their parents' working lives benefits children. She says, "I suppose I've taken this to an extreme; my 28-month-old son has been accompanying me to work since I returned to the office three months after his birth. It's been great on so many levels. I was able to breast-feed until we were both ready to stop; I have constant contact with my son and he with his mommy. He gets to experience different people coming into the office and see the way I interact with them, and he sees firsthand what I do—and now he can even help with some things!"

A landscape architect agrees that even young children can benefit from watching adults involved in productive work, "Children today are very isolated from the workplace. As a feminist, I have always thought that it was important for my children to see me at work. I have always brought them to meetings when I could, especially community meetings, so they will learn how to be involved in their community as they grow up." She adds, "My five-year-old, who is quite used to this, is very content to draw and color quietly and knows that Rule Number One is 'Don't interrupt Mommy when she's making a point!'"

Like the sons and daughters of farmers, shopkeepers, and other self-employed people through time, children who are integrated into their parent's working lives view themselves as more than dependents. They want to be partners in their parents' lifework, contributing as much as their age and abilities allow. For these children, taking on their own responsibilities is as natural as learning to walk. For their mothers, work is not something that takes them away from their children—and their children don't take them away from work.

Revising your picture of how work and mothering fit into your life can make as much of a difference as revamping the ways in which you work. Mentally dividing your life into separate spheres—mother, wife, worker, friend, and self (with separate standards of achievement for each)—could lead to despair and exhaustion. You may feel that you are falling short of your own high standards in every one of your roles, or that success in one means failure in another. Perfectionism, though it may have gotten you wherever you wanted to go in the past, will let you down now. So trade it in for flexibility. Let motherhood, beginning with breastfeeding, teach you not to juggle, shuffle, or balance working and mothering, but to *blend* them.

eight

CHANGING THE WORLD—
ONE NURSING, WORKING
MOTHER AT A TIME

*"I love my baby and I love my work.
Why does one always tear me from the other?"*

WHAT IS IT ABOUT WOMEN'S LIVES that stirs up controversy and intrusion? No matter the choices we make, the language we use, the paths we follow, there will be a stranger compelled to judge us. Perhaps no terms more than "working mother," "feminism," and, yes, "breastfeeding" attract more cold judgment of our personal lives.

When you head back out into the world newly cloaked in your status as a working mother and as a breastfeeding mother, you may find yourself suddenly in the center of several ongoing national debates. The headlines trumpeting this new finding on babies in daycare or that new discovery about breast milk may resonate more personally than ever before. The endless debate about the definition of feminism and whether mothers who work are leading the cause or burying it may thrust itself on you when you least expect it. "I'm just trying to take care of my baby, make my next deadline, and get more sleep," says one mother. "I really can't change the world, too, right now."

And yet, you are changing the world. Your expectation to be recognized for your vocational abilities without masking your identity as a mother, along with that of all the working women who were or are also engaged mothers, has changed our culture. Although we still have far to go, perhaps we are at last making headway to a more humanist society in which baby care and child raising (and caring for all our dependents, including the elderly) are freely performed by all of society's able members. When nurturing is esteemed equally with achievement, then the lives of mothers and children will become infinitely easier and more satisfying.

When we can employ our abilities publicly despite openly wearing this most womanly of emblems, motherhood, then feminism will truly have achieved its goals. Change begins with individuals. We can change the way our coworkers and managers perceive mothers in the workplace. Woman by woman, we can turn our culture into one that accepts the needs of children and enables all parents to meet those needs without penalty.

The first step is to dismiss any encounter that equates children with disruption, lack of productivity, and unprofessionalism. You begin to accomplish this when, instead of trying to make your baby as independent from you as possible, you ensure that your attachment is deep and secure. Breastfeeding and caring for your baby in the ancient ways of working mothers can help you stay close to him emotionally, and thus better able to meet his subtlest needs. And a child whose needs are met is far less likely to be disruptive when his parent must focus on something other than him. A well-attached child is generally easy to integrate into the adult world. He is not a distracting burden, but an amiable companion to his mother. The more you show this to the people you work with, the less threatened they will feel by your commitment to your child, the less convinced they will be that children and work do not mix.

Whether you bring your child into work daily, occasionally, or not at all, reject the notion that the image of a professional and the image of a mother are mutually exclusive. Be as open about your children and your life as a mother as you can be. You know that your role as a mother does not impair your ability to do well at work. Your coworkers will discover this too, if you let them. Find simple ways to remind them that you are a mother as much as an outstanding worker. Why not wear the bracelet your toddler made of pipe cleaners and plastic beads as part of your work attire? Frame your child's first work of art, and hang it alongside that diploma or award on your office wall or locker. Keep crayons and baby rattles in your desk for any child who comes into your workplace.

Do not allow your coworkers and managers—or yourself—to devalue that part of you that is a mother. Instead, apply in your working life the qualities that motherhood teaches—empathy, cooperation, flexibility, trust in your instincts, calmness in crises, respect for the irrational, the ability to do several things at once, and the ability to loosen control temporarily without losing control entirely.

Open channels between you and other mothers in your workplace. Change the social climate so that they too begin to feel that they can be open about their motherhood without compromising themselves professionally. Again, simple actions can initiate significant changes. Bring in a garment that your child has outgrown: "Can you use this? It's too small for Sammy, and I hate to throw it away." Ask about others' children. Ask new mothers how they're doing and if there is anything you can do to help. If coworkers grouse because someone has left early to pick up a child, point out how productive that person is and how little time she spends chatting at the water cooler. Share information about breastfeeding and pumping. Once women shared a common body of knowledge about mothering. Now even at-home mothers are often isolated from one another, and working mothers especially miss out on the rich exchange of support and advice that makes raising children comprehensible rather than bewildering. A network of working mothers in your company can substitute for a neighborhood or extended family network, if you do not have either of those in your life. Sharing your parenting concerns will help you all to work better and with more enthusiasm—while staying close to your children. (By all means include fathers in your network, but don't be surprised if they don't understand the daily challenges you face as fully as women do. Too many dads still don't manage the minutiae of their children's lives—packing extra clothes and diapers for daycare, remembering when daycare is closed, making substitute arrangements, etc.—or schedule doctor's appointments and play dates, much less pump and transport milk.)

If you can change the social climate so that parents feel free to support one another, the status of mothers in your workplace may change dramatically. A company is far more likely to institute benefits and options for employees with dependents if requested to do so by a united group of respected employees.

Companies that are truly family-friendly offer a range of ways to work besides the standard five-day-a-week, nine-to-five schedule. Many of these corporations are leaders in their fields, in part because their policies attract the best and brightest employees. As an executive at IBM writes, "Work-life issues are particularly important to our highest performers . . . [and] can have a direct positive impact on our ability to attract and retain a talented work force." Family-friendly policies are good for business.

When *Working Mother* magazine created its first list of family-friendly companies in 1986, the researchers found just 30 firms worth recognizing. Twenty years later, hundreds of employers compete to earn a spot on *Working Mother*'s list of the 100 best firms for employees with dependents.

What policies and benefits would be most helpful to you, and worth fighting for if they are not already in place in your company? A lactation station? Flextime? A "phase-back" policy to allow new mothers to return to the workplace gradually? The right to use your sick leave when your child is sick? How about a three- or four-month maternity leave? With pay, even? Other family-friendly benefits that could make a real difference in your life are "flexible spending accounts," pretax set-aside payroll programs (your child-care costs can be deducted from your pretax income and paid to you separately at year's end as an untaxed benefit), and reimbursement for child-care costs associated with business travel and overtime work. With a network of coworkers with children on your side, you may very well be able to realize your wish list of benefits in your workplace.

At home, if you have a spouse, his willingness to become an equal partner in running the household and caring for the children can do more than ease your workload. Your ability to give birth and breast-feed does not carry with it an extraordinary talent at grocery shopping and laundry. If both parents fully understand what it means to be a truly involved parent and to keep a home, both will also work to bring change to their workplaces. A vast change indeed is possible for our culture when individuals commit themselves to making it—and who is more committed than you, the nursing, working mother?

APPENDIX 1

BREASTFEEDING SUPPORT GROUPS

La Leche League International
1400 North Meacham Road
Schaumburg, Illinois 60173
800-LA-LECHE
847-591-7730
www.lalecheleague.org

Call between 9:00 A.M. and 5:00 P.M. CST for breastfeeding help or a referral to a local La Leche League group. Most local white pages list a La Leche League leader's phone number under "La Leche League."

Nursing Mothers Counsel, Inc.
P. O. Box 50063
Palo Alto, California 94303
408-291-8008
www.nursingmothers.org

Nursing Mothers Counsel has chapters in various cities in northern California. Call for a local number.

Boston Association for Childbirth Education (BACE)
Nursing Mothers' Council
P. O. Box 29
Newtonville, Massachusetts 02460
617-244-5102
www.bace-nmc.org

LACTATION CONSULTANT REFERRAL SERVICES

International Lactation Consultant Association
1500 Sunday Drive
Suite 102
Raleigh, North Carolina 27607
919-861-5577
www.ilca.org

Call weekdays between 9:00 A.M. and 5:00 P.M. EST, or visit
the ILCA Web site and click on "Find an International Board-
Certified Lactation Consultant in Your Area."

Breastfeeding National Network (Medela,Inc.)
800-TELL-YOU
www.medela.com

Call weekdays between 7:30 A.M. and 6:00 P.M. CST.

International Board of Lactation Consultant Examiners
7309 Arlington Boulevard, Suite 300
Falls Church, Virginia 22042
703-560-7330
www.iblce.org

Visit the organization's Web site and click on "U.S. regional
registry."

BREAST PUMP RENTAL INFORMATION

Medela, Inc.
P. O. Box 660
McHenry, Illinois 60051
800-TELL-YOU
www.medela.com

Call weekdays between 7:30 A.M. and 6:00 P.M. CST. Medela's
Breastfeeding National Network will refer you to a local rental
station where you can rent either a full-sized electric pump or the
more portable Lactina Plus, a lightweight, fully automatic pump.

Hollister Inc.
2000 Hollister Drive
Libertyville, Illinois 60048
800-323-4060

Call to locate a local rental station where you can rent either a
full-sized pump or the more portable Lact-E, a lightweight,
automatic pump.

HELPFUL WEB SITES FOR NURSING MOTHERS

www.breastfeeding.com

Information, support, and resources for nursing mothers.

www.breastfeedingonline.com

Information for nursing mothers.

www.kellymom.com

Information, products, and resources for nursing mothers.

www.motherlove.com

Personal care products for pregnant and nursing mothers.

www.pumpingmoms.org

Online discussion group for nursing moms who pump and store their milk.

www.bfar.org

Information for women who are breastfeeding after breast reduction.

www.fourfriends.com/abrw

Information for women who are or will be nursing adopted babies.

HELPFUL WEB SITES FOR WORKING MOTHERS

www.bluesuitmom.com

Information for professional working mothers and their employers concerning balancing work and family.

www.workingmother.com

Online version of *Working Mother* magazine, which covers work and life issues.

www.womensfinance.com

Financial planning advice and resources for women.

FAMILY AND WORK-LIFE ORGANIZATIONS

Families and Work Institute
267 Fifth Ave., Floor 2
New York, NY 10016
212-465-2044
www.familiesandwork.org

A nonprofit center for research on the changing work force, family, and community.

> The National Institutes of Health Work/Life Center
> www.wlc.od.nih.gov

The clearinghouse site for information on work/life resources for federal employees.

> Work & Family Connection
> 800-487-7898
> www.workfamily.com

Online work/life resources, news, and training.

> Catalyst
> 250 Park Avenue South, Fifth Floor
> New York, New York 10003
> 212-777-8900
> www.catalystwomen.org

A national nonprofit organization that works with businesses to effect change for women through research, advisory services, and publicity.

HOME-BASED BUSINESS RESOURCES

> Mothers Work at Home, Inc.
> www.mothersworkathome.com

This Web site provides information on starting a home business, with links to useful resources.

> Home-Based Working Moms
> www.hbwm.com

A professional association and online community of parents who work at home. Offers a directory of home-based careers and a weekly e-newsletter.

WAHM.com
www.wahm.com

An online magazine for work-at-home moms.

RECOMMENDED READING

Breastfeeding

Kathleen Huggins. *The Nursing Mother's Companion,* 5th ed. Boston: The Harvard Common Press, 2005.

Kathleen Huggins and Linda Ziedrich. *The Nursing Mother's Guide to Weaning,* 2nd ed. Boston: The Harvard Common Press, 2007.

La Leche League International. *The Womanly Art of Breastfeeding,* 7th ed. New York: Plume, 2004.

Karen Pryor and Gale Pryor. *Nursing Your Baby,* 4th ed. New York: HarperCollins, 2005.

Baby Care

Sharon Heller. *The Vital Touch : How Intimate Contact with Your Baby Leads to Happier, Healthier Development.* New York: Henry Holt, 1997.

Jean Liedloff. *The Continuum Concept: In Search of Happiness Lost.* Boston: Perseus Books, 1977.

Martha Sears. *25 Things Every New Mother Should Know.* Boston: The Harvard Common Press, 1995.

William Sears and Martha Sears. *The Baby Book: Everything You Need to Know about Your Baby from Birth to Age Two,* Rev. ed. Boston: Little, Brown, 2003.

William Sears, Robert Sears, and Martha Sears. *The Baby Sleep Book: The Complete Guide to a Good Night's Rest for the Whole Family.* Boston: Little, Brown, 2005.

Meredith Small. *Our Babies, Ourselves: How Biology and Culture Shape the Way We Parent.* New York: Random House, 1999.

Motherhood and Work

Katherine Ellison. *The Mommy Brain: How Motherhood Makes Us Smarter.* New York: Basic Books, 2005.

Linda Mason. *The Working Mother's Guide to Life: Strategies, Secrets, and Solutions.* New York: Crown, 2002.

Ann Pleshette Murphy. *The 7 Stages of Motherhood: Loving Your Life without Losing Your Mind.* New York: Anchor, 2006.

APPENDIX 2

Sample Proposal for Pumping Space

MEMO

TO: Human Resources Manager/Personnel Dept.

FR: Your name (or the names of all nursing mothers employed by your company)

RE: Proposal for accommodations for the use of working, nursing mothers

Currently, _____ staff members are the mothers of breastfed babies. In light of the number of women of childbearing age employed by [company name], it is likely that we will have more breastfeeding employees in the future. These employees each require a few minutes one to three times a day and an appropriate place in which to pump milk for their infants' meals during their separations due to work.

Pumping milk proceeds with more ease and is accomplished in significantly less time when it is done in a quiet, private space equipped with a few necessary items, including:

◆ a small room with a door that can be latched or locked from the inside;

◆ a comfortable chair and a small table;

◆ an electrical outlet within five to six feet of the table.

The following items are not necessary, but can enhance the usefulness of the room:

◆ a sink and a small refrigerator;

◆ a telephone for employees who would like to make or receive business calls while pumping their milk.

Facilities currently available to nursing mothers consist of the women's restroom, which is not an appropriately sanitary facility in which to prepare infant food; the employee locker room, which does not offer the privacy that speeds the pumping process; and borrowed private offices, which may inconvenience the primary users of these offices. A dedicated space for the use of nursing mothers will resolve all these problems.

Supporting breastfeeding mothers benefits the company in several important ways:

◆ Breastfed babies are statistically healthier babies. Healthy babies require that their parents miss fewer working days than do babies who have frequent respiratory and gastrointestinal illnesses. In addition, healthy babies mean fewer medical expenses for self-insured corporations such as [company name].

◆ Employees whose children are healthy and happy are better able to fully focus on their professional responsibilities.

◆ Employees who are able to pump plenty of milk at work (because a convenient, sanitary, and private pumping place has been provided) do not need to leave work in the course of the day to nurse their babies at daycare.

Support for nursing mothers is among the many diverse family-friendly benefits leading corporations across the country have instituted to secure a dedicated and loyal work force.

Thank you for your attention to this important issue. Please let me [us] know if you have any questions regarding this proposal.

SELECTED REFERENCES

American Academy of Pediatrics. "Statement on Breastfeeding." *Pediatrics* 115; 2, February 2005: 496-506.

Anderson, J. W., B. M. Johnstone, and D. T. Remley. "Breast-feeding and cognitive development: a meta-analysis." *American Journal of Clinical Nutrition,* 70; 4, 1999: 525-35.

Auerbach, K. G., and E. Guss. "Maternal employment and breast-feeding: A study of 567 women's experiences." *American Journal of Diseases of Children* 138, 1984: 958-60.

Baumslag, Naomi, and Dia L. Michels. *Milk, Money, and Madness: The Culture and Politics of Breastfeeding.* Westport, Connecticut: Bergin & Garvey, 1995.

Bettelheim, Bruno. *A Good Enough Parent: A Book on Child-rearing.* New York: Random House, 1987.

Bowlby, John. *Attachment and Loss,* Vol. 1. New York: Basic Books, 1969.

Clutton-Block, T. H. *The Evolution of Parental Care.* Princeton: Princeton University Press, 1991.

Driscoll, Jeanne, and Marsha Walker. *Taking Care of Your New Baby: A Guide to Infant Care.* Garden City Park, New York: Avery, 1989.

Edmond, Karen M., et al. "Delayed breastfeeding initiation increases risk of neonatal mortality." *Pediatrics* 117; 3, March 2006: 380-86.

Ehrenreich, Barbara, and Deirdre English. *For Her Own Good: 150 Years of the Experts' Advice to Women.* New York: Doubleday, 1978.

Ellison, Katherine. *The Mommy Brain: How Motherhood Makes Us Smarter.* New York: Basic Books, 2005.

Eibl-Eibesfeldt, Irenaus. *Human Ethology.* New York: Aldine de Gruyter, 1989.

Fildes, Valene. *Breasts, Bottles, and Babies.* Edinburgh: Edinburgh University Press, 1988.

Frantz, Kittie. *Breastfeeding Product Guide.* Sunland, California: Geddes Productions, 1994.

Greenspan, Stanley, M.D. *The Four-Thirds Solution: Solving the Childcare Crisis in America Today.* Boston: Perseus Books, 2001.

Hewlett, Sylvia Ann. *Creating a Life: Professional Women and the Quest for Children.* New York: Hyperion, 2002.

Hewlett, Sylvia Ann, and Cornel West. *The War Against Parents: What We Can Do for America's Beleaguered Moms and Dads.* Boston: Houghton Mifflin, 1998.

Hufton, Olwen. *The Prospect Before Her: A History of Women in Western Europe,* Vol. 1, 1500–1800. New York: Knopf, 1995.

Keith, Kristin, and Paula Malone. "Housework and the Wages of Young, Middle-Aged, and Older Workers." *Contemporary Economic Policy* 23; 2, 2005: 224-41.

Kennell, John H., and Marshall H. Klaus. *Parent-Infant Bonding,* 2nd ed. St. Louis: C. V. Mosby, 1982.

Kimbro, Rachel, Scott Lynch, and Sara McLanahan. "The Hispanic Paradox and Breastfeeding: Does Acculturation Matter? Evidence from the Fragile Families Study." Working paper, Center for Research on Child Wellbeing, Princeton University, 2004-01-FF.

Lawrence, Ruth A. *Breastfeeding: A Guide for the Medical Profession,* 2nd ed. St. Louis: C. V. Mosby, 1985.

Lawrence, Ruth A. "Breastfeeding" *(Clinics in Perinatology.* Vol. 14; No. 1*).* Philadelphia: W. B. Saunders, 1987.

Mohrbacher, Nancy, and Julie Stock. *The Breastfeeding Answer Book.* 3rd ed. Franklin Park, Illinois: La Leche League, 2003.

Neville, M. C., and M. R. Neifert, eds. *Lactation: Physiology, Nutrition, and Breastfeeding.* New York: Plenum Press, 1983.

Newton, Niles, with Michael Newton and others. *Newton on Breastfeeding: Reproductions of Early Classic Works.* Seattle: Birth and Life Bookstore, 1987.

Riordan, Jan. *A Practical Guide to Breastfeeding.* St. Louis: C. V. Mosby, 1983.

Riordan, Jan, and Kathleen G. Auerbach. *Breastfeeding and Human Lactation.* Boston: Jones and Bartlett, 1993.

Sears, William, and Martha Sears. *The Baby Book: Everything You Need to Know about Your Baby from Birth to Age Two,* Rev. ed. Boston: Little, Brown, 2003.

Saunders, Stephen, Julie M. Carroll, and Carol E. Johnson. *Breastfeeding: A Problem-Solving Manual,* 3rd ed. Dallas: Essential Medical Information Systems, 1990.

Tannen, Deborah. *Talking from 9 to 5: Women and Men in the Workplace: Language, Sex, and Power.* New York: Avon Books, 1994.

Thurer, Shari L. *The Myths of Motherhood: How Culture Reinvents the Good Mother.* Boston: Houghton Mifflin, 1994.

Ward, Mary J., and Elizabeth A. Carlson. "Associations among Adult Attachment Representations, Maternal Sensitivity, and Infant-Mother Attachment in a Sample of Adolescent Mothers." *Child Development* 66; 1, 1995: 69-79.

INDEX